PEDIATRIC EMERGENCY NURSING PROCEDURES

The Jones and Bartlett Series in Nursing

PEDIATRIC EMERGENCY NURSING PROCEDURES

EDITED BY

LISA MARIE BERNARDO, RN, MSN

Clinical Nurse Specialist
Children's Hospital of Pittsburgh
Pittsburgh, Pennsylvania

MARIANNE BOVE, RN, BSN, CEN

Clinical Nurse
Emergency Department
Children's Hospital of Pittsburgh
Pittsburgh, Pennsylvania

MEDICAL EDITOR

Raymond B. Karasic, M.D.

Associate Professor of Pediatrics
University of Pittsburgh School of Medicine
Staff Pediatrician
Emergency Department
Children's Hospital of Pittsburgh
Pittsburgh, Pennsylvania

MEDICAL ILLUSTRATOR

Eric Jablonowski

Jones and Bartlett Publishers
Boston   London

Editorial, Sales, and Customer Service Offices
Jones and Bartlett Publishers
One Exeter Plaza
Boston, MA 02116

Jones and Bartlett Publishers International
PO Box 1498
London W6 7RS
England

Library of Congress Cataloging-in-Publication Data

Pediatric emergency nursing procedures / edited by Lisa Maria
 Bernardo, Marianne Bove : medical editor, Raymond B. Karasic ;
 medical illustrator, Eric Jablonowski.
     p.   cm.
   Includes bibliographical references and index.
   ISBN 0-86720-330-7
   1. Pediatric emergencies.   2. Pediatric nursing.   I. Bernardo,
Lisa Maria.   II. Bove, Marianne.   III. Karasic, Raymond B.
   [DNLM: 1. Emergencies—in infancy & childhood.   2. Emergencies—
nursing.   3. Emergency Medicine—nurses' instruction.   4. Nursing
Process.   5. Pediatric Nursing—methods.   WY 159 P3693]
RJ370.P455   1993
618.92'0025—dc20
DNLM/DLC   91-18887
for Library of Congress   CIP

Printed in the United States of America
96 95 94 93 92   10 9 8 7 6 5 4 3 2 1

In memory of Margaret Miller, RN, MSED

CONTENTS

CONTRIBUTORS

Bonnie Clemence, RN, MSN
Charge Nurse
Emergency Department
Children's Hospital of Pittsburgh
Pittsburgh, Pennsylvania

Judith A. Conedera, RN, MSN, PNP
Nurse Practioner
Valparaiso, Indiana

Alice E. Conway, RN, PhD
Associate Professor
Graduate Nursing Program
Gannon University
Erie, Pennsylvania

Rita Ann Dello Stritto, RN, MSN, CEN, EMT-P
Charge/Staff Nurse
St. Luke's Episcopal Hospital
Texas Children's Hospital
Emergency Center
Houston, Texas

Stacey Lang, RN, BSN
Neurosurgical Nurse Coordinator
Department of Neurosurgery
Children's Hospital of Pittsburgh
Pittsburgh, Pennsylvania

Kathy MacPherson, RN, MA
Supervisor
Emergency Services
Kapiolani Medical Center for Women and Children
Honolulu, Hawaii

Linda Karen Manley, RN, BSN, CEN, CCRN
Pediatric Education Outreach Coordinator
Columbus Children's Hospital
Flight Nurse
SKYMED
Ohio State University Hospital
Columbus, Ohio

Sarah Martin, RN, MSN, CCRN
Pediatric Transplant Coordinator
University of Pittsburgh Medical Center
Pittsburgh, Pennsylvania

Kathleen O'Connor, RN, BSN
Education Specialist
Children's Hospital of Pittsburgh
Pittsburgh, Pennsylvania

REVIEWERS

Susan J. Kelley, RN, PhD, FAAN
Associate Professor
Maternal Child Health Graduate Program
Boston College School of Nursing
Chestnut Hill, Massachusetts

Becky Martin, RN, BSN, CEN
Clinical Educator
Emergency Department
Providence Hospital
Everett, Washington

C. Richard Packer, MS, NREMT-P
Prehospital Care Coordinator
Saint Margaret Memorial Hospital
Pittsburgh, Pennsylvania

Laura Skidmore Rhodes, RN, MSN
State Board of Nurse Examiners
Charleston, West Virginia

Margery Samsel, RN, MSN, CCRN
Education Coordinator
Special Care Services
Harrisburg Hospital
Harrisburg, Pennsylvania

Donna Ojanen Thomas, RN, MSN, CEN
Nursing Director
Emergency Department
Primary Children's Hospital
Salt Lake City, Utah

William Welsh, RN, MSN, CEN
Humana Hospital System
Cleveland, Ohio

PREFACE

Thirty percent of the 86,000,000 annual visits to emergency departments are by children.[1] These children are brought to the emergency department by their parents or guardians for treatment of emergent, urgent, and nonurgent health conditions. The emergency nurse must be adept at recognizing the emergently ill or injured child and performing appropriate nursing interventions.

Emergency nurses who do not routinely perform procedures on children feel uncomfortable or ill prepared when asked to do so. This book was written to assist these nurses in preparing children and families for procedures as well as to offer suggestions on how to best perform these procedures.

Pediatric Emergency Nursing Procedures focuses on procedures routinely or infrequently performed on children in the emergency department. The text begins with two chapters on the physical and psychosocial assessment of children. The next chapter describes immobilization (restraining) techniques. Subsequent chapters organize procedures according to a systems approach. The remaining chapters describe the administration of medications and the collection of evidence for suspected physical and sexual abuse.

Each procedure follows an organized format. The procedure's indications and contraindications are outlined, followed by potential complications. The required equipment list gives recommended sizes for children of each age group. Next, psychosocial considerations are presented to guide the nurse in assisting the child and family to understand and to cope with the procedure. Finally, the nursing actions and rationale are detailed in a two-column format. References are included at the end of each chapter.

Before performing any procedure in this text, emergency nurses should review their state's Nurse Practice Act, as well as their hospital's policy and procedure manual. Most importantly, universal precautions should always be maintained.

REFERENCE
1. ACEP News, January 1990.

ACKNOWLEDGMENTS

The completion of this text was possible through the dedication and support of many individuals. The chapter authors deserve our gratitude for sharing their expertise. Raymond Karasic, MD, provided much clinical and editorial assistance. Eric Jablonowski created the detailed illustrations, while Laura Dugan and Norman D. Rabinovitz provided the medical photography. Their efforts are gratefully acknowledged. Mag Clutter provided skillful manuscript preparation. The reviewers supplied honest and thoughtful critiques.

The models for this book deserve mention for their patient endurance during the photography sessions. They are Mrs. Judith Conedera and her children Paul, Carl, and Laura; Ms. Edith Green and her son, Eugene Wellon; and Mrs. Carole Shepard and her daughter, Maureen.

Finally, the efforts of Angela Gladfelter, our Production Coordinator from York Production Services, and John Servideo from Jones and Bartlett who took this project to completion are gratefully acknowledged.

Quick Reference to Pediatric Emergency Equipment*

EQUIPMENT / AGE	PREMATURE	NEONATE	6 MONS.	1 Y	2 Y	3 Y	4 Y	5 Y	6 Y	7 Y	8 Y	9 Y	10 Y	11-18 Y
Airway														
Oral airway[1] (size)	Infant	Infant/ Small	Small	Small	Small	Small	Med	Med	Med	Med	Med/ Lg	Med/ Lg	Med/ Lg	Large
Endotracheal tube[2] (mm) * = cuffed	2.5-3.0	3.0-3.5	3.5-4.0	4.0-4.5	4.0-4.5	4.0-4.5	5.0-5.5	5.0-5.5	5.5-6.0	5.5-6.0	6.0*- 6.5*	6.0*- 6.5*	6.0*- 6.5*	7.0*- 8.0*
Laryngoscope blade[1] s = straight c = curved	0 s	1 s	1 s	1 s	1 s	1 s	2 s/c	2 s/c	2 s/c	2 s/c	2-3 s/c	2-3 s/c	2-3 s/c	3 s/c
Suction catheter[2] (French)	5	6	6	8	8	8	10	10	10	10	10	10	10	12
Breathing														
Face mask[1] (size)	Premie NB	NB	NB	Ped	Ped	Ped	Ped	Ped	Ped	Ped	Ad	Ad	Ad	Ad
Bag-valve device[1] (size)	Inf	Inf	Inf	Ped	Ped	Ped	Ped	Ped	Ped	Ped/Ad	Ad	Ad	Ad	Ad
Chest tube[1] (French)	10-14	12-18	14-20	14-24	14-24	14-24	20-32	20-32	20-32	20-32	28-38	28-38	28-38	28-38
Circulation														
Over-the-needle catheter[3] (gauge)	22-24	22-24	22-24	20-22	20-22	20-22	20-22	18-22	18-20	18-20	16-20	16-20	16-20	14-18
Intraosseous device (gauge)	18	15	15	15	15	15	15	15	–	–	–	–	–	–
Gastrointestinal/ Genitourinary														
Nasogastric tube[4] (French)	5	5	8	8	10	10	10	10	10	12	12	12	12	14-16
Urinary catheter[1] (French)	5 feeding tube	5-8 feeding tube	8	10	10	10	10-12	10-12	10-12	10-12	12	12	12	12-18

[1]Committee on Trauma. Advanced Trauma Life Support Student Manual. Chicago: American College of Surgeons, 1989; 231.

[2]Motoyama E. Endotracheal intubation. In Motoyama E. and Davis P. (eds) Smith's Anesthesia for Infants and Children. St. Louis: CV Mosby Co., 1990; 275.

[3]Chameides L. Ed. Textbook of Pediatric Advanced Life Support. Dallas: American Heart Association and American Academy of Pediatrics, 1988; 35:105.

[4]Skale N. Manual of Pediatric Nursing Procedures. Philadelphia: JB Lippincott Co., 1992; 407.

*This reference demonstrates suggested sizes only. Always consider each child's size and health condition when selecting appropriate equipment for procedures.

1

Physical Assessment and Triage

Judith Conedera

INTRODUCTION

The accurate assessment and recognition of a seriously ill or injured child occurs during triage. Triage addresses those aspects of the history and physical assessment that are of immediate priority in determining the child's disposition in the emergency department. This chapter describes (a) ways to gain the child's and the parent's cooperation, (b) prioritized history-taking, and (c) physical assessment approaches.

GAINING THE CHILD'S AND THE PARENT'S COOPERATION

An understanding of normal developmental characteristics is essential when interacting with children of any age (see Chapter 2 "Psychosocial Assessment"). Suggested interventions for gaining cooperation of the child and parent are listed in Tables 1.1 and 1.2.

While a relaxed, calm demeanor helps in gaining the trust of the child and parent, organization and skill are also necessary to expedite the triage process. Age-specific approaches to physical assessment are outlined in Table 1.3.

PRIORITIES IN OBTAINING A HEALTH HISTORY

The emergency nurse relies on the parents or guardians to provide an accurate history of their child's present illness or injury. Parents know their child best, and their perceptions of the child's condition must be respected.

Questions to ask about the child's health history include

Length of current illness—How long has the child been coughing, vomiting, having diarrhea, pulling at ears?

Table 1.1.   Ways to Gain the Child's Cooperation

INTERVENTION	RATIONALE
1. Show a genuine interest in the child; ask about hobbies, likes, dislikes, pets, and so on.	Helps the child begin to trust you; shows that you respect the child as a person.
2. Address the child by name.	Demonstrates that you consider her or him as an individual and not, for example, just a "child with a fractured arm."
3. Allow time for the child to adjust to the emergency department environment before proceeding with the history and physical assessment.	Rushing into a history and assessment without building up trust may hinder further efforts at eliciting information.
4. Protect the child's privacy. Avoid performing a physical assessment or obtaining a history in the waiting area.	Lack of privacy hinders the establishment of trust and may make the child feel vulnerable and exposed.
5. Warm your hands and equipment prior to the physical assessment; keep the room at a warm temperature.	Promotes comfort.
6. Listen to what the child has to tell you.	Helps to gain the child's trust; provides information.

Table 1.2.   Ways to Gain the Parent's Cooperation

INTERVENTION	RATIONALE
1. Address the parent by name.	Demonstrates that you are considering the parent as an individual.
2. Allow time for the parent to talk about the child's health problem.	Rushing into a history and assessment without listening to the parent may hinder your efforts and may cause the parent to withhold important information.
3. Protect the parent's privacy by asking health or financial information in a private area.	Asking such questions in a crowded waiting area creates a feeling of vulnerability.

Circumstances surrounding the injury—How did the injury occur? Was there a loss of consciousness? What was the type of injury?

Child's general condition—What has the child been doing at home? Is the child eating, eliminating? How much? How frequent?

Exposure to chicken pox—Has the child been exposed?

Have any home remedies or remedial measures been taken at home?

Current medications—Is the child currently taking any? When were they last given?

Known allergies—Does the child have any?

Ongoing health conditions (congenital heart disease [CHD], chronic illnesses, organ transplant)

Table 1.3. Age-Specific Approaches to Physical Assessment

INFANT

INTERVENTION	RATIONALE
1. Seat the infant on the parent's lap or against the parent's shoulder.	Helps the infant feel secure.
2. Always save the most intrusive aspects of the assessment for last (e.g., rectal temperature).	Allows for more accurate measurement of heart and respiratory rates; decreases anxiety.
3. Measure the infant's blood pressure, temperature, and heart and respiratory rates with the infant held against the parent's shoulder.	Promotes comfort and security.
4. Speak in soft tones.	Calms the infant.
5. Use nonsense ("baby") talk.	Distracts the infant.
6. Avoid quick movements.	Avoids surp.ises.
7. Avoid prolonged eye contact with older infants.	Promotes trust.

TODDLER

INTERVENTION	RATIONALE
1. Allow the toddler to remain in the parent's lap or upright against the parent's body while obtaining the blood pressure, temperature, and heart and respiratory rates.	Promotes trust and comfort.
2. Always save the most intrusive aspects of the assessment for last (e.g., rectal temperature).	Allows for more accurate measurement of heart and respiratory rates; decreases anxiety.
3. Allow the child to hold his or her transitional object or favorite toy during the assessment.	Helps child develop trust in the environment.
4. Speak to the child in terms that a toddler can understand.	Helps child understand what will happen next.
5. Keep the parent's face in the child's view as much as possible.	Promotes security and decreases fear of abandonment.
6. In difficult situations, decide what has to be accomplished, and help the child get through the physical assessment as quickly as possible.	Avoids distress and confrontation.

PRESCHOOLER

INTERVENTION	RATIONALE
1. Always save the most intrusive aspects of the assessment for last (e.g., rectal temperature).	Allows for more accurate measurement of heart and respiratory rates; decreases anxiety.

Table 1.3. (*cont.*)

PRESCHOOLER	
INTERVENTION	RATIONALE
2. Allow the child to handle equipment, such as the stethoscope or thermometer.	Helps to promote sense of exploration.
3. Talk to the child and explain in simple, feeling terms why you need to assess his or her body. Ask for the child's help whenever possible, such as pointing to the area that hurts, holding the blood pressure cuff, and so forth.	Decreases anxiety and helps to gain cooperation.
4. Use this time to educate the child about his or her body. ("I am going to listen to your heart. Can you point to your heart. What does your heart do for you?")	Promotes health teaching and allows time to clarify misconceptions.

SCHOOL-AGE	
INTERVENTION	RATIONALE
1. Talk to the child in terms that he or she can understand about what you will be doing.	Lessens anxiety; information seeking is a way of maintaining control.
2. Ask the child how he or she feels; tell the child that it is okay to cry.	Encourages expression of feelings.
3. Maintain privacy at all times, especially during any disrobing.	Respects need for privacy and may help to lessen anxiety regarding potentially intrusive procedures.

ADOLESCENT	
INTERVENTION	RATIONALE
1. Speak to the adolescent first prior to talking with the parents. Obtain health history information from the child.	Respects the adolescent as an individual.
2. Respect the adolescent's need or desire for parental presence, and allow the adolescent to choose his or her support person.	Recognizes need for the adolescent to make own choices.
3. Explain all procedures and why they are being performed.	Decreases anxiety; the adolescent has a more advanced understanding of body structure and function.
4. Maintain privacy during assessment and procedures.	Minimizes the adolescent's insecurities due to rapidly changing body image. Offers the adolescent a sense of personal control.

Immunization status — Have immunizations been provided regularly? How recently were they updated?

Who is the child's pediatrician or primary health-care provider?

PHYSICAL ASSESSMENT APPROACHES

A detailed assessment should be performed each time the child visits a health-care facility. During triage, however, the nurse first addresses those aspects of the physical assessment that are of immediate priority (airway, breathing, circulation, and neurological status). This section focuses only on these priorities; a comprehensive approach to pediatric physical assessment can be found in numerous nursing texts.[1,2]

Much of the physical assessment done at triage is accomplished by observation. The additional "hands-on" assessment validates the nurse's observations.

Assessment Parameter	Variations in the Pediatric Assessment	Abnormal Findings Requiring Immediate Attention
Airway		
Observe the airway for patency. Listen for any abnormal sounds (cough, stridor, snoring). Observe the child's position during breathing ("sniffing" position, refusal to lie flat). Be alert to malodorous breath. Note the child's ability to swallow. Note any nasal discharge (color, amount, consistency, and crusting).	Children with obstructive breathing due to nasal congestion or enlarged adenoids usually have adequate aeration. Drooling may be a usual state for infants and children who are teething. Children's lower airways are smaller, and the supporting cartilage is less developed, as compared to the adult; airway obstruction can easily occur from mucus, blood, pus, edema, and so on.[3]	The "sniffing" position, refusal to lie flat, and drooling are indicative of epiglottitis. Malodorous breath and/or inability to swallow may indicate a chemical ingestion or peritonsilar abscess. Inability to swallow is also seen with an upper-airway esophageal foreign-body obstruction. Obstruction of the nose or nasopharynx causes snoring or snorting sounds (stertor).[4] Laryngeal and subglottic obstruction usually manifests with high-pitched inspiratory stridor; expiratory wheezes are usually heard with bronchial obstruction.[4] Inspiratory and expiratory stridor are present with tracheal obstruction and may also be seen with a high esophageal foreign-body obstruction.[4]

Assessment Parameter	Variations in the Pediatric Assessment	Abnormal Findings Requiring Immediate Attention
Breathing		
1. Observe the child's respiratory pattern. Note the child's work of breathing. Observe for retractions, wheezing, grunting, nasal flaring, head bobbing. Note any asymmetrical chest movement, use of accessory muscles, respiratory effort, and rate and depth of respirations.	Due to higher oxygen demands and metabolic rates, respirations in children are faster than those of adults. In infants and young children, diaphragmatic breathing predominates.[1] In older children, breathing becomes thoracic. In infants, the normal chest shape is round; it assumes a more oval shape with growth.	Retractions that are intercostal, suprasternal, substernal, supraclavicular, subclavicular, or intraabdominal ("seesaw") indicate varying levels of respiratory distress. Expiratory wheezing is indicative of lower-airway obstruction. Nasal flaring and head bobbing are related to air hunger. Asymmetrical chest movement may be the result of a lower-airway foreign-body obstruction or of pneumonia, pneumothorax, or atelectasis.
2. Auscultate the child's breath sounds with the child quiet (optimal situation) (Figure 1.1). Assess breath sounds for pitch, intensity, quality, location,	Because the hemithorax of an infant or child is very thin, the breath sounds are easily transmitted from one side to the other. The breath sounds therefore	Adventitious sounds (crackles, rubs, rales, rhonchi, wheezing) or absent breath sounds are indicative of lung pathology. A hoarse cry or voice indicates pos-

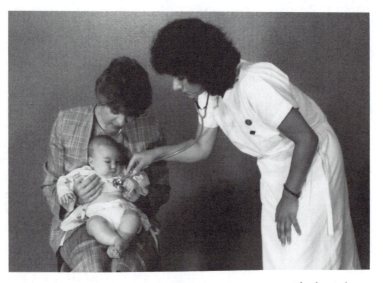

Figure 1.1. Performing a respiratory assessment with the infant in the mother's lap. Note the infant's interest in the environment.

| Assessment Parameter | Variations in the Pediatric Assessment | Abnormal Findings Requiring Immediate Attention |

and duration. Note any adventitious sounds. Measure the child's respiratory rate. Note the quality and tone of crying or talking.

sound louder and harsher than those in adults because the stethoscope is placed closer to the origin of the sounds.[1] Auscultation of the infant's chest is done using the bell or the small diaphragm of the stethoscope to allow for localization of the findings.[1] See Table 1.4 for normal vital signs.

sible upper airway obstruction. A cephalic (high-pitched) cry is indicative of central nervous system (CNS) infection or injury. Respiratory rates that are above or below the normal range for the child's age indicate need for further evaluation, (if the rates are not associated with crying).

Circulation

1. Observe the color of the skin (pallor, cyanosis, dusky, mottling) and mucous membranes.

Pallor and mottling represent poor peripheral perfusion. A dusky or cyanotic color means inadequate tissue oxygenation; however, a child with CHD normally may have this appearance. Pale skin and/or mucous membranes may indicate a low hemoglobin.

2. Auscultate the apical heart rate at the point of maximal impulse (PMI) while the child is quiet (optimal situation). Note the rate, rhythm, quality of heart tones, and presence of murmurs.

In children with thin chest walls, the PMI might be seen or felt as a slight pulsation. The PMI should be at the level of the fourth intercostal space until age 7 years, when it drops to the fifth intercostal space.[1]

Muffled, distant, or diffused heart tones indicate pathology. A heart rate that is lower or higher than the normal range for the child's age requires further evaluation. Failure to feel the PMI or marked dis-

Table 1.4. Vital Signs by Age [a]

AGE	RESPIRATIONS	PULSE	BLOOD PRESSURE Systolic
Newborn	30–60	100–160	50–70
1–6 Wks.	30–60	100–160	70–95
6 Months	25–40	90–120	80–100
1 Year	20–30	90–120	80–100
3 Years	20–30	80–120	80–110
6 Years	18–25	70–110	80–110
10 Years	15–20	60–90	90–120

[a] From Seidel JS and Henderson DP, eds. Prehospital pediatric emergencies. Los Angeles: Pediatric Society California Chapter 2 American Academy of Pediatrics, 1987:10, reprinted with permission.

Assessment Parameter	Variations in the Pediatric Assessment	Abnormal Findings Requiring Immediate Attention
	Murmurs may be present and are either innocent or organic. An *innocent murmur* is heard in the absence of cardiac disease.[1] An *organic murmur* is associated with CHD or acquired heart disease.[1] In children, slight speeding of the heart during inspiration and slowing during expiration (sinus arrhythmia) can occur and is normal. The heart rate should be the same as the radial pulse. See Table 1.4 for normal vital signs.	placement of the PMI may indicate a pneumothorax or pneumomediastinum.
3. Check for capillary refill, and palpate for peripheral pulses. Obtain a blood pressure.		Capillary refill of longer than 2 seconds indicates poor peripheral perfusion.

Neurological Status

1. Observe the child's activity level (playful, withdrawn, inactive, lethargic). Note muscle tone (e.g., floppy). Observe the parent–child interaction. Note any seizure activity (lip smacking, eye deviations, tremors). Observe for (a) asymmetry in gait and muscle strength, (b) poor balance, and (c) muscle tone.	Adequacy of neurological functioning is determined by these parameters. Seizure activity may be subtle, due to the infant's or young child's immature neurological system.	A quiet, withdrawn child who does not make eye contact should be investigated for suspected physical or sexual abuse. An inactive, disinterested child may have an underlying pathology (ingestion, sepsis, CNS trauma); an overactive child should lead to the suspicion of an ingestion. Problems with gait, muscle strength and tone, and balance can signify inadequate cerebellar functioning. Inability to respond to stimulation and/or paradoxical irritability indicates CNS involvement.
2. Palpate the anterior fontanel while the infant is quiet and sitting or held in	The anterior fontanel closes between 4 and 26 months; the posterior fon-	A bulging, full anterior fontanel indicates increased intracranial pressure;[1] a

Assessment Parameter

an upright position.[1] Ascertain nuchal rigidity in the older child.

3. Ask the child simple, direct questions to ascertain the level of consciousness. Note pupil size and shape, as well as equality of the pupils.

Other Parameters

Temperature

Obtain a temperature (rectal, oral, axillary, tympanic).

Weight

Obtain the child's weight; dress the infant or child lightly (diaper, patient gown).

Skin

1. Observe for petechial bruising, purpura, infectious diseases (varicella, measles, impetigo, jaundice).

2. Test skin turgor; observe for sunken eyes, dry mucous membranes.

Variations in the Pediatric Assessment

tanel closes by 2 months.[1]

Older infants who are fed yellow vegetables may have a pale yellow-orange skin color (carotenemia), which is limited to the soles, palms, nose, and nasolabial folds.[1]

Abnormal Findings Requiring Immediate Attention

depressed fontanel indicates dehydration. Nuchal rigidity suggests meningeal irritation.

Inability to recognize parents or familiar objects indicates CNS pathology. Unequal pupils indicate third-cranial-nerve involvement.

In infants younger than 3 months of age, temperatures over 101°F or subnormal temperatures indicate the possibility of sepsis.

Loss of weight in a short period of time may indicate dehydration. Children who fall below the weight range for their age and/or who appear emaciated or cachexic should be investigated for child maltreatment.

Either petechiae below the chest or purpura suggests septicemia. Unexplained bruising suggests potential child abuse (see Chapter 13) or possible coagulopathies. Infectious or contagious diseases require isolation measures.

Poor skin turgor, sunken eyes, dry lips and mucous membranes, and decreased urine output indicate dehydration.

Table 1.5. SAVE-A-CHILD, Recognition of the Seriously Ill Pediatric Patient

Skin	Mottled? Cyanotic? Petechiae? Pallor?
Activity	Needs assistance? Not ambulating? Responsive?
Ventilation	Retractions? Head bobbing? Drooling? Nasal flaring? Slow rate? Fast rate? Stridor? Wheezing?
Eye contact	Glassy stare? Fails to engage/focus?
Abuse	Unexplained bruising/injuries? Inappropriate parental behavior?
Cry	High-pitched or cephalic? Irritable?
Heat	High fever (>41 degrees)? Hypothermia (<36 degrees)?
Immune system	Sickle cell? AIDS? Corticosteroids?
Level of con- sciousness	Irritable? Lethargic? Pain only? Convulsing? Unresponsive?
Dehydration	Hollow eyes? Capillary refill? Cold hands, feet? Voiding? Severe diarrhea? Vomiting: projectile, bilious, persistent? Dry mucous membranes?

Source: Prepared by the Aloha Chapter, Hawaii Emergency Nurses Association, 1990, reprinted with permission.

Note: SAVE: Observations made prior to touching the child.
  CHILD: History from caregiver and brief exam.

One concise approach to the triage of the pediatric patient is the SAVE-A-CHILD method. This approach combines history and physical assessment parameters to recognize the seriously ill child. The SAVE-A-CHILD method is outlined in Table 1.5.

A systematic, prioritized approach to assessing the child in the emergency department provides the emergency nurse with the means to identify the critically ill child and to intervene accordingly.

REFERENCES
1. Hoekelman RA. The physical examination of infants and children. In: Bates B, ed. A guide to physical examination and history taking, 5th ed. Philadelphia: JB Lippincott, 1991:561–.
2. Thompson SW. Emergency care of children. Boston: Jones & Bartlett Publishers, 1990:1–34.
3. Chaemeides L, ed. Textbook of pediatric advanced life support. Dallas: American Heart Association, American Academy of Pediatrics, 1988:21.
4. Handler SD. Stridor. In: Fleisher G and Ludwig S, eds. Textbook of pediatric emergency medicine, 2nd ed. Baltimore: Williams & Wilkins, 1988:300–301.

2

Psychosocial Considerations for the Child and Family

Alice E. Conway

PSYCHOSOCIAL CONSIDERATIONS WITH THE CHILD IN THE EMERGENCY DEPARTMENT

A visit to the emergency department can be a frightening experience for a child of any age. Nursing interventions, based on principles of psychosocial growth and development, facilitate children's and adolescents' coping abilities before, during, and after emergency nursing procedures.

Three recommendations when performing emergency nursing procedures with children are:

1. Call the child by name. This action shows respect for the child as a person.
2. Each child is a unique individual, with an identifiable personality and temperament, as well as specific needs. Guidelines of development are only that, and they should not be substituted for individualized care.
3. Most children come to the emergency department with their family. However, if the family is not present, one emergency nurse should remain with the child to serve as an advocate and support person until the family's arrival.

A variety of health-care professionals is available to assist emergency nurses with preparing, assisting, and comforting children before, during, and after procedures. These professionals are pediatric clinical nurse specialists, child life specialists, child psychologists and psychiatrists, and child development experts.

INFANTS (BIRTH TO 12 MONTHS)[1]

Infants depend on others to meet their needs. The essential tasks of infancy are formation of a stable emotional bond with the parent and development of a sense of trust.[1] If the infant's basic needs are not met in a consistent manner, he or she develops a sense of mistrust that affects subsequent stages of development.[1]

Hallmarks of infancy relevant to emergency nurses are as follows:

At about 8 months, infants respond to unfamiliar people with anxiety.[2] This phenomenon is known as separation anxiety. See Figure 2.1.

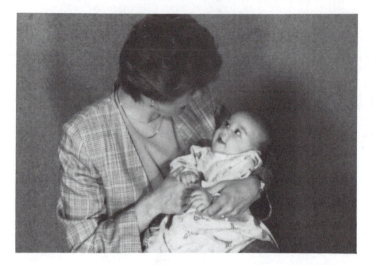

Figure 2.1. Parent–infant interaction. Note how the infant responds to the mother's facial expression. Before, during, and after emergency procedures, try to keep infants with their parents or at least have the parents stay in sight.

Infants are able to feel pain. There is evidence that the pain pathways and cortical centers required for pain perception and the neurochemical systems associated with pain transmission are present and functional in both preterm and term newborns.[3]

Tables 2.1, 2.2, and 2.3 list nursing interventions to help infants before, during, and after emergency nursing procedures.

Table 2.1.   Nursing Interventions to Prepare Infants for Procedures

NURSING ACTIONS	RATIONALE
1. Warm your hands and keep the room warm.	Infants are sensitive to the physical environment.[4]
2. Perform nursing assessments and interventions with the infant seated upright on the parent's lap, as appropriate.	Decreases separation; provides security and comfort.
3. Keep the infant with the parent, or at least have the parent stay in sight as much as possible (see Figure 2.1).	Visual contact with the mother promotes maternal attachment and provides security and comfort.[5]
4. Consider sedatives or analgesics, if needed.	Newborns and infants have all of the physiological mechanisms necessary to perceive pain.[6]

Table 2.2. Nursing Interventions to Assist Infants During Procedures

NURSING ACTIONS	RATIONALE
1. Talk softly to the infant and keep the environmental activity level quiet.	Provides comfort and distraction as infants are fascinated with sounds.[7]
2. Offer self-comforting opportunities, such as using a pacifier or positioning the young infant with the legs flexed and the hands near midline or close to the mouth. When possible, refrain from immobilizing the hand the infant prefers to suck.	Sucking provides comfort through the oral cavity and allows the infant to provide self-comfort.
3. Allow rest periods between procedures.	Large amounts of energy are expended during illness, injury, and painful procedures. Napping restores energy; when overwhelmed, the infant withdraws into sleep.[8]
4. Observe for pain behaviors, such as increased pulse, respiration, and blood pressure; body tenseness; and high-pitched, prolonged, rhythmic, and perhaps broken crying. Facial expressions of grimacing, fear, or vigilance, and thrashing or pulling away are also indications of pain behavior in infants.[9]	

Table 2.3. Nursing Interventions to Comfort Infants After Procedures

NURSING ACTIONS	RATIONALE
1. Release the infant as soon as the procedure is completed.	Infants diffuse stress and frustration through motor activity.[10]
2. Reunite the parent and infant; encourage the parent to comfort the infant through swaddling, rocking, holding, and touching.	Decreases anxiety due to separation; promotes trust.

TODDLERS (1 TO 3 YEARS)[1]

Increasing motor and language skills are characteristics of toddlers. These skills allow the toddler to become an active explorer of self, others, and the environment. The toddler is developing a sense of autonomy, and the parents struggle with the toddler's need for control and assertive declarations ("Me do it," "No!"). Failure to achieve autonomy leads to shame and doubt.[11] Should this occur, the toddler withdraws and is unable to test limits and thus does not learn about self and about the environment.

Hallmarks of toddlerhood relevant to emergency nurses are:

Toddlers must separate themselves from their families to experience autonomy. While necessary, this separation can cause fears. The toddler copes with these fears by clinging, withdrawing, regressing, being aggressive, and using a transitional object (security blanket).

Between 18 and 24 months of age, toddlers are capable of determining a cause after observing an effect within the limits of their prior experience[12] (e.g., going to the emergency department may mean an injection that hurts).

Toddlers have a poor concept of time, especially the future, but they understand time in terms of a daily schedule (e.g., "Daddy will be home after your nap").

Toddlers possess limited expressive-language skills, understanding more than they are able to verbalize. Toddlers focus their attention for a short time period.

Toddlers are learning to control their bodies and are developing fears about it being harmed. They respond to painful events by hitting, kicking, biting, and teeth clenching. While toddlers can localize the pain ("leg hurts"),[13] they cannot yet describe the intensity or type of pain.

Tables 2.4, 2.5, and 2.6 list nursing interventions to help toddlers before, during, and after emergency procedures.

PRESCHOOLERS (3 TO 5 YEARS)[1]

As children leave the toddler years, they move into the preschool years, the stage of initiative. If children's initiative is not rewarded at this stage, or if children are not allowed to feel good about what they can do, a sense of guilt may develop. Children with this sense of guilt restrict their activities and exploration, develop a sense of failure and "badness," and fantasize about others harming them.[11] Hallmarks of preschoolers relevant to emergency nurses are

Preschoolers eagerly explore everyone and everything. The boundaries between make-believe and reality easily blur. A primitive sense of right and wrong develops, and they try hard to please others. While preschoolers have a sepa-

Table 2.4.   Nursing Interventions to Prepare Toddlers for Procedures

NURSING ACTIONS	RATIONALE
1. When possible, approach the child slowly and gradually. Hold out your hand or a toy as an introduction, and talk to the child and the parent.	Minimizes stranger anxiety. Shows that the parent accepts you as a safe stranger.
2. Perform the nursing assessment and interventions with the child seated in an upright position if possible.	Helps the child feel less vulnerable than when in a supine position.[14]
3. Keep on the child's eye level—bend down, sit, squat. Be alert to how equipment looks from the child's viewpoint.	A new environment reminds children of their own smallness and lack of control.[15]
4. Consider sedatives or analgesics, if needed.	Decreases pain; promotes comfort.

Table 2.5. Nursing Interventions to Assist Toddlers During Procedures

NURSING ACTIONS	RATIONALE
1. Explain to the toddler in simple, concrete words what the toddler will feel during the procedure just immediately before the procedure begins. Offer choices, when appropriate.	Shows sensitivity to children's fear of harm to their bodies.[16] Toddlers' language ability is limited. The child's concept of time is not well developed.
2. Tell the child, "I will help you."	Helps the child to gain control. A means of coping is to accept help.[17]
3. If the parent is not present, give the child a token item from the parent or the child's own transitional object.	Provides comfort for the child and decreases the child's sense of separation.[18,19]
4. Allow a moderate amount of verbal and motor protesting.	Motility is the child's best avenue of handling his anger.[15]
5. Give the toddler something to hold, such as a Band-aid™ or tape.	Promotes autonomy, sense of control, and self-respect.[20]
6. Allow choices when possible.	Helps the child feel less threatened.
7. Involve the parent as much as possible.	Reduces the child's fear of separation and abandonment.[18,19]
8. If the child is upset or anxious, divert the child's attention through games and toys, then proceed as quickly as possible.	The toddler's emotions are freely expressed, and the toddler has limited internal controls.
9. Observe for pain behaviors, such as crying, whimpering, thrashing, verbalization ("head hurts").	

Table 2.6. Nursing Interventions to Comfort Toddlers After Procedures

NURSING ACTIONS	RATIONALE
1. Release any securing device as quickly as possible.	Avoids prolonged anxiety.
2. Give praise freely, and provide a positive experience after the procedure, such as a drink of juice or a Popsicle™, if appropriate. Give a sticker as a reward.	Praise enhances the child's self-esteem.[20] When offered a positive experience afterwards, the toddler remembers a positive health-care experience.
3. Never imply that the child was bad.	Minimizes the older toddler's tendency to perceive pain as punishment for wrongdoing.[20]
4. Reunite the toddler and the parent. Allow the parent to comfort the child.	Decreases anxiety due to separation; promotes comfort.

rate identity from that of their parents, they need their parents to reassure, set limits, and prevent loss of control.

Young preschoolers remain egocentric and believe that others view the world the same way they do.

Preschoolers believe that pain is punishment for "bad" or angry thoughts or actions. Thus, the preschooler whose strong inquisitiveness led to an injury and a visit to the emergency department believes that he or she is being punished for this inquisitiveness.

Sex-typing and sex-role identification is the major task of this developmental stage.

Preschoolers fear bodily intrusions. Therefore, measuring a rectal temperature is almost as traumatic as an injection.

Preschoolers possess better developed language skills and can describe the location and the intensity of their pain.[13] They use language skills to avoid painful procedures ("Wait until my Mommy comes," "I'll be good if you don't give me a shot").[13]

Tables 2.7, 2.8, and 2.9 list nursing interventions to help preschoolers before, during, and after emergency procedures.

SCHOOL-AGE CHILDREN (6 TO 12 YEARS)[1]

The school-age child enters the psychosocial stage of industry; school-age children eagerly apply themselves to tasks that will win approval.[11] If the child does not gain approval and instead experiences repeated rejection and failure, a sense of inferiority develops that stunts further psychosocial growth.[11] Hallmarks of school-age children relevant to emergency nurses are

School-age children less than 7 years of age are able to reason only on the basis of one characteristic at a time.[25] For example, they can recognize the relationship

Table 2.7. Nursing Interventions to Prepare Preschoolers for Procedures

NURSING ACTIONS	RATIONALE
1. Encourage verbal expression of fears. Ask about any previous hospital experiences.	Permits the nurse to clarify any misconceptions. Egocentric thinking leads the child to believe he or she is being punished for a real or imagined wrongdoing.[22] The preschool child believes that events closely following one another have a cause–effect relationship.[21] Guilt combined with fantasy creates erroneous impressions and causes generalized fears.[11]
2. Allow the child to explore the equipment or to use the equipment on a doll. Show the child how the equipment works.	Decreases the child's reported fantasies; direct action is a means of coping.[17]
3. Consider sedatives or analgesics, if needed.	

Table 2.8.   Nursing Interventions to Assist Preschoolers During Procedures

NURSING ACTIONS	RATIONALE
1. Explain to the preschooler in simple, concrete words the need for the procedure. Include sensations that the child may experience, such as *cold, wet, pinch*.[20]	Avoids any unexpected sensations that might otherwise increase anxiety and may cause the child to lose trust. When the child is told what sensations he or she may feel, the amount of distress associated with pain decreases.[20]
2. Allow a minimal time lapse between the explanations and the procedure.	Avoid long time lags, during which younger children frighten themselves with imagined horrors.[22]
3. Use non-threatening language, such as *fix, repair, check, sore, uncomfortable*.	Minimizes children's fear of invasive procedures. These words are descriptive and arouse more manageable feelings than such words as *cut*, or *opening*.[22]
4. Acknowledge the child's feelings and reassure the child that it is okay to be scared or upset. Give suggestions to help the child master these feelings, such as "hold my hand," "say ouch if it hurts," "let's take some deep breaths together."	Increases the child's control over emotions, which are heightened by stress, and promotes the child's sense of mastery.
5. Allow the child's parents to participate. Offer the child choices, when appropriate.	Minimizes children's natural fear of separation, especially during a crisis.[20]
6. Watch for the child's use of behaviors that prolong the onset of a procedure, such as verbal stalling, crying, fighting, making excuses, and bargaining.	These actions are direct coping mechanisms used by preschool children.[17]
7. Reinforce the child's coping behaviors: "You are such a big help."	Reinforcement of the child's efforts helps avoid instilling a sense of failure in the child. Promotes the child's emotional growth.
8. Allow the child to participate in the procedure by holding a Band-aid™ or tape, if the child desires to do so.	Promotes a sense of competence and provides positive reinforcement.
9. Observe for masked pain behaviors, such as guarding a body area, withdrawal, decreased activity, and even sleep.	Because the preschoolers' fear of injections is great, they may try to mask their pain to avoid receiving an injection.
10. Provide measures for pain relief, such as guided imagery,[4] storytelling, hypnosis.[4,23] Use a pain scale to help the child evaluate his or her pain.	Minimizes preschoolers' fears about mutilation and pain related to their belief that their skin holds them in. Preschoolers are more interested in their body surfaces than older children.[24]

Table 2.9.   Nursing Interventions to Comfort Preschoolers After Procedures

NURSING ACTIONS	RATIONALE
1. Release the preschooler from any securing device as soon as possible; reunite the child with the parent.	Avoids prolonged anxiety.
2. Reward the child with praise and stickers after the procedure. Offer drinks of juice or Popsicles™, if permitted.	Allows for mastery.
3. Use Band-aids™ liberally.	Recognizes the child's concern for body intactness and vulnerability (a small scratch is a big issue).[15]

between a single cause of illness (e.g., germs) and getting sick. Between the ages of 7 and 11 years, the child can take note of several features and their interrelationships instead of focusing on only one feature.[25]

School-age children possess an expanding vocabulary, a full understanding of time, and increasing cognitive abilities. However, school-age children still attribute illness as punishment for their actions and are confused about the function of internal organs with the illness experience.

School-age children shift from a family-oriented environment to a peer-dominated society.[26] Older children may wish to manage without their parents present; however, if stressed, these children may need to have their parents available. When feeling threatened, as in an emergency situation, school-age children may withdraw and become reserved instead of seeking information.

School-age children are interested in the insides of their bodies, and are determined to learn about their bodily functions and limitations.[27] Bodily injury, loss of body functions, loss of control, and loss of status are major worries and fears of this age group.[20]

School-age children are able to describe the intensity, duration, and location of their pain.

Tables 2.10, 2.11, and 2.12 list nursing interventions to help school-age children, before, during, and after procedures.

ADOLESCENTS (13 TO 19 YEARS)[1]

Adolescence is characterized by a myriad of interacting biological, emotional, and social challenges. The adolescent experiences conflicts associated with the search for a personal identity, separation from the family, establishment of peer-group relationships, management of sexual feelings,[30] and future career choices.[28] Central to all of these experiences is the effort to develop a unique personal identity that they carry into adulthood.[11] Over time, the adolescent develops his or her own individual identity and makes choices on the basis of stable personal values. If a personal identity is not achieved, role confusion or diffusion occurs, leading to an excessive identification with others, persistent dependence on others, and a lack of self-confidence.[11]

Hallmarks of adolescence relevant to emergency nurses are:

Adolescents are able to take into account all of the variables within a situation. They become idealistic and are egocentric when considering their ideals in

Table 2.10. Nursing Interventions to Prepare School-Age Children for Procedures

NURSING ACTIONS	RATIONALE
1. Use anatomical models and equipment to explain the procedure.	Concretizes body organs and processes.[16] Takes advantage of the child's cognitive abilities.
2. Prepare for the procedure with enough time for the child to formulate questions.	Recognizes that asking questions is a major way in which the school-age child copes.[17]
3. If the child asks no questions, yet looks anxious, provide an open-ended statement to draw out his or her concerns. "Some children ask about getting stitches [e.g.], would you like to know this information, too?"	Provides a means for the child to turn an inhibition-or-action mechanism into a direct-action mechanism, thereby increasing his or her ability to cope.[17]
4. Assess how the child has coped with past procedures or stressful situations.[13] If previous coping behaviors were ineffective, give the child concrete examples of how to cope, such as positioning or deep breathing.	Increases the child's emotional and developmental growth (sense of industry).
5. State the approximate length of the procedure, but be as accurate as possible. Five more minutes should not turn into 15 minutes.	School-age children have a concept of past, present and future.[20]
6. Consider sedatives or analgesics, if needed.	

Table 2.11. Nursing Interventions to Assist School-Age Children During Procedures

NURSING ACTIONS	RATIONALE
1. Offer choices about care and about how to proceed.	Helps the child to feel in control.
2. If possible, encourage the child to participate in the care.	Conveys a sense of control and decreases the child's dependence.
3. Allow the parent to be present; encourage the parent to help the child to cope; permit siblings or friends to visit the child if appropriate.	Serves as a support system for the child.
4. Provide distraction during the procedure; offer storytelling, counting, relaxation techniques. If possible, practice these techniques prior to the procedure.	These direct-action techniques minimize passive resistance, such as clenched fists or teeth and body rigidity.[13]

Table 2.11.   (*cont.*)

NURSING ACTIONS	RATIONALE
5. If the child is struggling to maintain control, offer suggestions; praise the child's efforts, and minimize attention to losing control.	School-age children's locus of control is becoming more internal than external. They have overly high and sometimes unrealistic expectations of themselves.[28]
6. Maintain a positive manner regardless of the child's reaction.	Prevents feelings of inferiority and decreased self-esteem.
7. Project a positive outcome.	Minimizes school-age children's fears of disfigurement and responds to their incomplete understanding of death.[4]
8. Observe for pain behaviors through passive resistance (clenched fists or teeth, body rigidity, regression). Use a pain rating scale.	In order not to lose status, the school-age child may deny feeling pain during a procedure.[13] Allows for assessment of pain severity.[29]

Table 2.12.   Nursing Interventions to Comfort School-Age Children After Procedures

NURSING ACTIONS	RATIONALE
1. Praise the child for completing the procedure.	Provides positive reinforcement.
2. Reunite the child with the family.	Offers a support system.
3. Encourage the child to talk about his or her experience of the procedure.	Allows verbalization of feelings; affords the opportunity to clarify any misconceptions.

relation to those of others in the world.[25] Due to this idealism and their introspection, they are very critical of their own appearance and behavior, and they think that others are equally focused on them.

Adolescents understand causes of health and illness in physiological terms, and alternative health behaviors and their consequences are explored. Respecting the adolescents' independence and values will increase chances of cooperation. Adolescents should be able to understand the risks and consequences associated with certain behaviors. Some of these risk taking behaviors, such as active experimentation with alcohol and other drugs, may impair the adolescent's ability to make wise choices about his or her health.[30]

Peers are especially important, and independence from parents is a major theme. Ill or injured adolescents may regress and want their parents present. This, however, is highly individual.

Adolescents experience uncertainty about themselves as persons and about whether their bodies, thoughts, and feelings are normal.[30] Ill or injured adolescents fear loss of autonomy, privacy, and peer acceptance and have concerns about death. Adolescents are particularly sensitive to the way others perceive them.

Tables 2.13, 2.14, and 2.15 list nursing interventions to help adolescents, before, during, and after procedures.

Table 2.13.   Nursing Interventions to Prepare Adolescents for Procedures

NURSING ACTIONS	RATIONALE
1. Talk with the adolescent first before talking with the parents.	Demonstrates respect for the adolescent as an individual with a developing sense of self-identity. Also, adolescents want to be part of the decision-making about their own bodies and health care.
2. Provide health information to the adolescent. Explain the procedure, using appropriate anatomical and physiological terminology. Use a textbook or a model.	Recognizes that adolescents can use reason and logical thinking and that information-seeking is a major way of coping.[17] Shows sensitivity to the adolescent's more advanced understanding of body functions and ability to use abstract thought.[20] Acknowledges that adolescents are curious about anything that affects them and that they need reassurance that they are normal.[30]
3. Provide opportunities for choices and control. For example, ask which arm or leg they prefer for an injection or intravenous insertion.	Promotes the adolescent's self-esteem.[28]
4. Consider sedatives or analgesics, if needed.	

Table 2.14.   Nursing Interventions to Assist Adolescents During Procedures

NURSING ACTIONS	RATIONALE
1. Ensure and maintain privacy during the procedure. Use gowns and drapes to promote modesty. Tell the adolescent what to expect before touching him or her.[30]	Recognizes that body image concerns are heightened during adolescence, due to increased hormonal, physical, and emotional changes, resulting in heightened sensitivity toward personal appearance.[31] Respecting physical modesty and autonomy and allowing choices and control facilitates cooperation.[32]
2. Allow the adolescent to choose a support person to remain with him or her.	Demonstrates sensitivity to the adolescent's need or desire for parental presence.
3. Promote the adolescent's autonomy and incorporate the adolescent in decision-making.	Decreases the adolescent's loss of autonomy.[32]
4. Encourage the adolescent to verbalize anger, frustration, and fear, but suggest coping strategies and redirect the adolescent's energies.	Adolescents have language skills necessary to verbalize their feelings. Rebellion is often part of adolescence when loss of control is perceived. Demonstrates the nurse's calm, nonjudgmental approach.

Table 2.14. *(cont.)*

NURSING ACTIONS	RATIONALE
5. Provide coping strategies, such as music, deep breathing, guided imagery, along with appropriate analgesia.	Aids in coping with stressful procedures and helps adolescents to maintain control.
6. Observe for signs of masked pain behavior, such as grimacing or denying the pain.	

Table 2.15.   Nursing Interventions to Comfort Adolescents After Procedures

NURSING ACTIONS	RATIONALE
1. Reunite the adolescent with the family or other support persons after the procedure.	
2. Reconfirm the adolescent's normalcy; when possible, allow a peer to be a support person.	Acknowledges that the peer group can be more important to an adolescent than the family.[28]
3. When appropriate, reassure adolescents that they will get better; accept their questions.	Responds to the adolescent's fear of death and developing sense that death is permanent.[33]

PSYCHOSOCIAL CONSIDERATIONS FOR THE FAMILY IN THE EMERGENCY DEPARTMENT

The families of today are complex and diverse. The two-parent biological family is no longer the norm. Children live with single parents, step families, foster families, and host families. Children are adopted or are conceived through nontraditional means. Families' cultural, ethnic, racial, religious, minority, and alternative life-style needs must be recognized and respected. This text interchanges *parents* and *families* in recognition of this diversity.

Parental participation during procedures is guided by a number of factors. These factors include:

a . The urgency of the situation.
b. The invasiveness of the procedure.
c . The staff's comfort in performing the procedure in the family's presence.
d. The availability of a health professional to stay with the family exclusively during the procedure.
e . Written hospital policies, procedures, or standards of care addressing parental participation.
f . The family's ability to support and comfort the child during the procedure.

The presence of siblings during procedures is also individualized and is guided by a number of factors. These factors include:

a . The sibling's age and developmental abilities.

b. The urgency of the situation.

c . The invasiveness of the procedure.

d. The staff's comfort in performing the procedure in the sibling's presence.

e . The availability of a health professional and family member to stay with the sibling exclusively during the procedure.

f . Written hospital policies, procedures, or standards of care addressing sibling participation.

Three recommendations useful when interacting with families are:

1. Try to keep the family and child together. Encourage the family to participate in the child's care if they demonstrate a willingness to do so and are able to support the child adequately.

2. Keep the family informed of their child's treatment at frequent intervals. A designated health-care professional should perform this function to build a trusting relationship with the family.

3. Each family, like each child, is unique. Guidelines are just that, and should not be substituted for individualized care.

Tables 2.16, 2.17, and 2.18 list nursing interventions to help families cope when their child undergoes an emergency procedure.

Table 2.16.   Nursing Interventions to Prepare Families for Procedures

NURSING ACTIONS	RATIONALE
1. Provide information in a factual, concrete, and timely manner. Let parents know that you realize the difficulty of waiting.	Waiting is a major stressor for families.[34] Providing information can help families to cope.[35]
2. Assess how the parents interact with the child, to determine the parent-child relationship.	If parents demean the child, it is not helpful to have them assist with the procedure or examination.
3. Ask the family about the child's previous health-care experiences and how the child responded. Specifically ask what coping strategies the child has used in the past.	Demonstrates to the parents their importance as information givers and initiates your relationship with them.
4. Have the parents identify a support person for themselves or call a health-care professional who can provide support.	Acknowledges that parents also need support and allows the emergency nurses to spend their energy and time with the child.
5. If the child arrives in the emergency department before the parents, prepare the parents for how the child appears.	Parents feel extreme anxiety and are often shocked by their child's appearance; preparation can lessen the shock.[36]
6. Maintain a calm, nonjudgmental approach.	Families may respond to their child's injury or illness with seemingly irrational emotions, such as anger.[37]

Table 2.17.   Nursing Interventions to Assist Families During Procedures

NURSING ACTIONS	RATIONALE
1. Tell the child's parents, prior to their participation in a procedure, that you may ask them to leave, depending on how the child is responding or how they themselves are responding.	Establishes an honest relationship and informs the parents that you have their child's best interest as a priority.
2. If the parent does not remain for the procedure, ask the parent for one of his or her belongings for the child to hold.	Maintains the participation of the parent and reassures the child that the parent will not abandon him or her.
3. If the parent is present for the procedure, have the parent provide emotional support to the child.	Allows the parent to contribute positively to the situation. For infants: Get close to the infant's face, and talk in a soothing voice so the infant will maintain contact with the parent's face; provide a pacifier. For toddlers: Stroke the toddler's forehead, hold the child's hand, speak quietly, and tell a story; reassure the child that it is acceptable to cry but he or she must remain still. For preschoolers: Take deep breaths together, use a party blower, tell a story, and have the child contribute to a section of the story.[13,38,39] For school-age children: Use guided imagery or relaxation techniques; tell the child how long he or she needs to hold still; encourage positive self-talk such as "I can make it."[39] For adolescents: Allow adolescents to decide whom they want present during the procedure; ask how they want to get through the procedure such as "What helped you before when you had this procedure done to you?"
4. If the parents make statements that seem to demonstrate unrealistic expectations of the child, provide a realistic explanation of what a child of that age might be expected to do.	Provides appropriate information about child development and about how children may respond to stressful events. Prevents censure of the child.
5. Suggest to parents some positive approaches to assisting the child. Serve as a role model.	Actively incorporating parents in the care of their child helps them to maintain their parenting role. Focuses the parents' energies on their strengths and maximizes their positive adaptation to the situation.

Table 2.17.   (cont.)

NURSING ACTIONS	RATIONALE
6. If the procedure is lengthy or the parents appear to have reached the end of their endurance, provide respite for them.	Shows respect for parents as individuals with strengths and limitations.
7. Assist the parents to use coping strategies that have helped them in other stressful situations. Consider using relaxation techniques or providing information.	Children, particularly the very young, pick up on their parents' anxiety and become more anxious themselves[39] (emotional contagion theory).

Table 2.18.   Nursing Interventions to Support Families After Procedures

NURSING ACTIONS	RATIONALE
1. Encourage the parent to comfort the child after the procedure if the parent is able to do so.	Promotes parent-child interaction.
2. Ensure the availability of additional resources as needed (clergy, social services, home health care, community shelters, crisis centers, etc.).	Promotes continuity of care.
3. Alert the family to postdischarge behaviors the child might exhibit. These behaviors include temporary sleep and feeding difficulties; regressive behavior, such as bed-wetting or clinging, in young children; rebellious behavior in older children.[40] The child may also play "emergency room". Play is frequently a means by which children gain mastery over a stressful experience. Tell parents to remain patient, reassure the child, and discuss the emergency experience in simple, honest terms to clarify the child's misconceptions.[41]	These behaviors are generally temporary and short-lived. If the behaviors continue, the parents should discuss them with their primary health-care professional.

REFERENCES

1. Wright M, D'Antonio I, Servonsky J. Application of theories of psychosocial development. In: Servonsky J, Opas S, eds. Nursing management of children. Boston: Jones & Bartlett, 1987:266–267, 269, 271–272, 274.
2. Skerret K, Harden S, Puskar K. Infant anxiety. Matern Child Nurs J 1983; 12:54.
3. Anand K, Hickey P. Pain and its effect on the human, neonate, and fetus. N Engl J Med 1987; 317:1326.

4. Selbst S, Henretig F. The treatment of pain in the emergency department. Pediatr Clin North Am 1989; 36:968–969.

5. Mercer R. Parent–infant attachment. In: Sonstegard L, Kowalski K, Jennings B, eds. Women's health: Childbearing. Vol. II. New York: Grune & Stratton, 1987:21.

6. Porter F. Pain in the newborn. Clin Perinatol 1989; 16:550.

7. Aslin R. Visual and auditory development in infancy. In: Osofsky L, ed. Handbook of infant development. 2nd ed. New York: John Wiley, 1987:66–67.

8. Brazelton TB. Appendix. Commentary 3. In: Gottfried A, Gaiter J, eds. Infant stress under intensive care. Baltimore: University Park Press, 1985:281.

9. Mills N. Pain behaviors in infants and toddlers. J Pain Sympt Manage 1989; 4:187.

10. Kulka A, Fry C, Goldstein F. Kinesthetic needs in infancy. Am J Orthopsychiatry 1960; 30:562.

11. Erikson E. Childhood and society. 2nd ed. New York: W.W. Norton, 1963:85, 256, 259–262.

12. Piaget J, Helder S. The psychology of the child. New York: Basic Books, 1969:24.

13. Lutz W. Helping hospitalized children and their parents cope with painful procedures. J Pediatr Nurs 1986; 1:25–26, 28, 30.

14. Bernardo L, Conway A, Bove M. The ABC method of emotional assessment and intervention: A new approach in pediatric emergency care. J Emerg Nurs 1990; 16:73.

15. Erickson F. Helping the sick child maintain behavioral control. Nurs Clin North Am 1967; 2:697, 702.

16. Pidgeon V. Characteristics of children's thinking and implications for health teaching. Matern Child Nurs J 1977; 6:6.

17. Ritchie J, Caty S, Ellerton M. Coping behaviors of hospitalized preschool children. Matern Child Nurs J 1988; 17:159, 163–164, 167.

18. Winnicott D. Mother and child. New York: Basic Books, 1957:183.

19. Wear R. Separation anxiety reconsidered: Nursing implications. Matern Child Nurs J 1974; 3:14.

20. Pridham K, Adelson F, Hansen M. Helping children deal with procedures in a clinic setting: A developmental approach. J Pediatr Nurs 1987; 2:15–21.

21. Bibace C, Walsh M. Development of children's concepts of illness. Pediatrics 1980; 66:914.

22. Goldberger J, Gaynard L, Wolfer J. Helping children cope with health-care procedures. Contemp Pediatr 1990; 7:153–154.

23. Eland J. Pain in children. Nurs Clin North Am 1990; 25:881.

24. Anthony J. The child's discovery of his body. Phys Ther 1968; 12:1109.

25. Maier H. Three theories of child development. 3rd ed. New York: Harper & Row, 1978:54, 56.

26. Scarr S, Weinberg R, Levine A. Understanding development. New York: Harcourt Brace Jovanovich, 1986:423.

27. Levine M, Carey W, Crocker A, Gross R. Developmental behavioral pediatrics. Philadelphia: W.B. Saunders, 1983:112.

28. Gottlieb M, Williams J. Self-concept in the latency period and adolescence. Feelings and their medical significance. Columbus, OH: Ross Laboratories, 1982; 24:23.

29. McGrath P. Pain in children: Nature, assessment, and treatment. New York: The Guilford Press, 1990:78.

30. Manning M. Health assessment of the early adolescent. Nurs Clin North Am 1990; 25:827, 829.

31. Riddle I. Nursing intervention to promote body image integrity in children. Nurs Clin North Am 1972; 7:659.
32. Denholm C, Ferguson R. Strategies to promote the developmental needs of hospitalized adolescents. Child Health Care 1987; 15:184–185.
33. Gordon AK. The tattered cloak of immortality. In: Corr C, McNeil J, eds. Adolescence and death. New York: Springer Publishing, 1986:20.
34. Savedra M, Tesler M, Ritchie J. Parents' waiting: Is it an inevitable part of the hospital experience? J Pediatr Nurs 1987; 2:329.
35. Gillis C, Rose D, Hallburg J, Martinson I. The family and chronic illness. In: Gillis C, Highley B, Roberts B, Martinson I, eds. Toward a science of family nursing. Reading, MA: Addison-Wesley, 1989:295.
36. Lewandowski L. Stresses and coping styles of parents of children undergoing open heart surgery. Crit Care Q 1980; 3:78.
37. Solurshi D. The family of the trauma victim. Nurs Clin North Am 1990; 25:158.
38. Hunsberger M, Love B, Byrne C. A review of current approaches used to help children and parents cope with health care procedures. Matern Child Nurs J 1984; 13:160.
39. Melamed B, Ridley-Johnson R. Psychological preparation of families for hospitalization. J Dev Behav Pediatr 1988; 9:98, 100.
40. Fletcher B. Psychological upset in post-hospitalized children: A review of the literature. Matern Child Nurs J 1981; 10:186.
41. Association for the Care of Children's Health. Caring for your child in the emergency room. Washington, D.C.: The Association, 1989:13.

3

Positioning and Securing Children for Procedures

Marianne Bove

Performing invasive procedures on children requires dexterity and skill. Success in cannulating an infant's vein, for example, is in part determined by the positioning and securing of the child during catheter insertion. *Positioning* of the child involves placing the child in a position conducive to completing the procedure. *Securing* the child involves keeping the child still during the procedure, through human, physical, or pharmaceutical means.

Emergency nurses must keep in mind the psychological effects of securing modalities on the child. Lying in a supine position and being secured by people or devices is very frightening for the child. The child's fright causes her or him to struggle more, which increases the parents' anxiety; the parents then may take out their anxiety and frustration on the emergency staff. To avoid the potential for escalating the child's and parents' emotions, explain the purpose for securing the child prior to the procedure. Position and secure the child before the procedure begins; stopping the procedure because the child is afraid and uncooperative only prolongs the procedure and heightens the anxiety. Do not assume that the young child will be able to lie still for a procedure requiring "only about 15 minutes," such as minor suturing. Young children have no concept of time, and to them, it seems like "forever" that they are requested to remain still. If possible and appropriate, have the parent talk to the child during the procedure, offering words of encouragement and support. This action helps both the parents and the child to cope during the procedure.

GUIDELINES FOR POSITIONING AND SECURING CHILDREN

1. Position the child properly before the procedure begins.
2. Hold the child securely for procedures requiring a few minutes to complete, such as IV insertion or lumbar puncture. If more attempts are needed, give the child a

rest between attempts, to avoid depleting the child's energy stores. Never have the parent restrain the child, as the child will feel betrayed.

3. Secure the child in a mummy restraint or a papoose board for procedures requiring a fair to moderate amount of time, such as suturing, or eye or ear irrigations. The nurse holding the child, as well as the child, will quickly become fatigued, making further attempts to proceed impossible.

4. Sedate the child for procedures that are painful or uncomfortable, or that require a prolonged amount of time such as closed reductions, or extensive suturing. It is not fair to the child to be restrained in a device for an extended period of time. Sedation helps to minimize the psychological trauma of the procedure, as well as to minimize the child's pain and discomfort. If sedation is used, have resuscitative equipment and trained personnel readily available.

5. Use age-appropriate coping techniques, as outlined in Chapter 2, to minimize anxiety during procedures.

PAPOOSE BOARD

Indications   The papoose board is used with young children who are not voluntarily able to hold still for procedures requiring a fair to moderate amount of time, such as suturing, eye and ear irrigations, or foreign body removal.

Contraindications   The papoose board (or any other restraining device) is never used as a substitute for more appropriate measures.[1]

Complications   Potential for aspiration, from vomiting. Uncommon complications are bruising, vascular compromise and child mistrust.[2]

Equipment Needed

> 1 sheet
> 1 papoose board
>   small (infants and toddlers)
>   large (preschool and small school age)

Psychosocial Considerations   Children feel vulnerable and threatened when they are restrained, which makes them struggle even more. Explain to children that the board will give them a "hug." Allow children to wiggle their hands or feet during the procedure to provide them with some mobility. Have the parent sit at the child's head in a direct line of vision so that the child can see the parent. Encourage the parent to talk to the child, stroke the child's hair, and so forth, to provide comfort. Tell the child what will happen so that the child can anticipate and prepare for what he or she will experience.

In regard to nursing responsibilities, see Table 3.1.

Table 3.1. Nursing Responsibilities

INTERVENTION	RATIONALE
1. Explain the need for the papoose board to the child and the family.	Enhances their understanding and cooperation.
2. Place the papoose board on the stretcher, with the velcro straps opened. Place a sheet in a triangular fashion over the papoose board.	

Table 3.1. *(cont.)*

INTERVENTION	RATIONALE
3. Have the child lie supine on the board, with her or his arms down at each side. Bring the right corner of the sheet over the child's body and tuck it under the child's left arm and torso; repeat for the other side. (See Figure 3.1(a).)	Secures the child properly.
4. Place the Velcro® straps snugly over the child. (See Figure 3.1(b).) If the child is struggling and wiggling, open the straps, and readjust the sheet; additional assistance may be required.	Keeps the child secure.
5. Allow the child to move a body part, such as feet or hands, during the procedure.	Allows for some mobility and control.
6. When the procedure is completed, remove the child as soon as possible.	Allows the child to regain some control.
7. Praise the child for being cooperative.	Gives the child a sense of mastery over the situation.
8. Methods for positioning and securing without the papoose board are demonstrated in Figures 3.2 and 3.3. See Chapter 6 (Procedures Involving the Cardiovascular System) and Chapter 8 (Procedures Involving the Neurological System) for additional securing techniques.	Allows for alternative modes of positioning and securing the child.

Figure 3.1. Sequence for restraining a child with a papoose board. **(a)** Place a sheet on the papoose board in a triangular fashion. Have the child lie with arms at sides. Bring one corner of the sheet across the child's body and tuck it under the arm and torso.

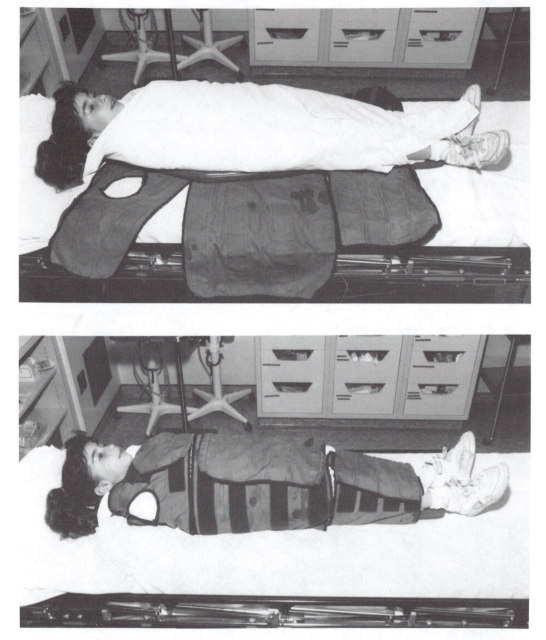

Figure 3.1. *(cont.)* **(b)** Repeat this procedure for the other side, making sure that the child is snug without compromising respiratory effort. **(c)** Fasten the Velcro straps over the child's chest, abdomen, and legs. Because the child may be frightened by being immobile, allow some movement (wiggling toes, flexing feet, etc.).

Figure 3.3. Positioning the young child in the left lateral decubitus position for a lumbar puncture. Note how the nurse is able to observe the child's reactions, as well as to provide emotional support verbally. An alternative method is to place the left arm beneath the child's thighs and to grasp his or her wrists—this action restrains both the arms and the legs.

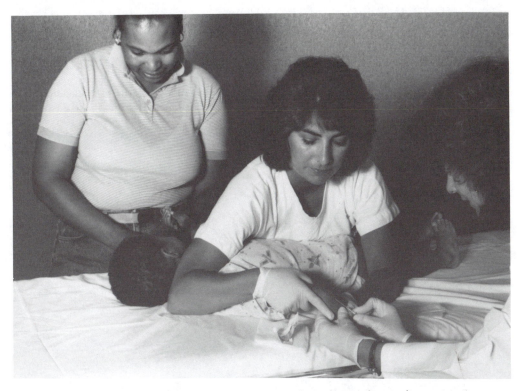

Figure 3.2. Holding the child for IV insertion. Note how the mother is distracting the child; his head is turned away from the insertion site. The "holding" nurse is able to immobilize the child's body by leaning over him, supporting her weight on her arms. She is then able to hold the extremity for cannulation.

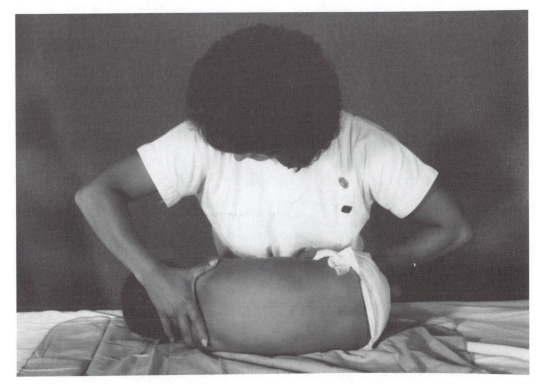

REFERENCES
1. Waechter EH, Phillips J, Holaday B. Nursing care of children. 10th ed. Philadelphia: JB Lippincott, 1985; 1401.
2. Cohen DE, Broennle AM. Emergency department anesthetic management. In Fleisher G and Ludwig S, eds. Textbook of pediatric emergency medicine. 2nd ed. Baltimore: Williams & Wilkins, 1988; 54.

4

Procedures Involving the Airway

Linda Karen Manley

OVERVIEW OF PEDIATRIC AIRWAY DIFFERENCES

Airway obstruction resulting in hypoxia is almost always the precipitating event in a pediatric cardiopulmonary arrest.[1-11] Choking is a leading cause of accidental death in young children, especially in those under the age of 5 years.[6] Commonly aspirated objects include hot dogs, round candies, nuts, balloons, grapes, raw carrots, and popcorn. Complete airway obstruction may also be the result of an infectious disease, such as epiglottitis or croup. Children with an infectious etiology, however, need prompt attention in an advanced life-support facility rather than a futile and dangerous attempt to relieve this type of airway obstruction.[5,6]

Nurses caring for infants and children must be aware of the anatomical airway differences in children, as compared with adults, (Table 4.1) and must be proficient with various airway maneuvers and equipment. Evaluation of the child's airway has the highest priority. Small air passages can easily be obstructed with blood, mucus, vomitus, or—in the unconscious child—the tongue. Often, a basic airway maneuver is all that is needed to provide a patent airway.

OPENING THE AIRWAY

Chin Lift

Indications   The chin lift is used in the infant or child with poor respiratory effort and/or signs of airway obstruction, with possible cervical spine injury.

Contraindications   None.

Complications   None.

Table 4.1.   Differences in Airway: Adult Versus Child[1,3]

ANATOMICAL FEATURE	ADULT	PEDIATRIC
Size of tongue in proportion to oral cavity	Smaller	Larger
Larynx	Cylindrical, located at C6	Funnel-shaped, located at C3 (more cephalad), more anterior
Epiglottis	Flatter	Shorter, U-shaped in the infant, and more mobile
Oral Cavity		Gums soft, vascular, and easily indented; deciduous teeth poorly anchored and easily dislodged
Cricoid Cartilage	Firm cartilage support	Soft, lacks cartilage support
Smallest diameter	Vocal cords	Cricoid cartilage
Results of 1-mm edema at cricoid ring	Airway reduction of 19%	Airway reduction of 50–75%

Equipment

> Small towel
> Gloves

Psychosocial considerations   This procedure is performed on the child with an altered level of consciousness. Speak to the child in a calm and soothing voice, as if she or he were fully conscious. Keep the family apprised of the child's treatment; if they choose to remain in the room, have a support person stay with them to tend to their needs.

Nursing responsibilities are described in Table 4.2.

Head Tilt

Indications   The head-tilt method is used in the infant or child with poor respiratory effort and/or indications of airway obstruction where the potential for cervical spine injury does *not* exist. It is often used in conjunction with the chin-lift maneuver and in the unconscious child.

Contraindications   Any possibility of head or spinal cord trauma.

Complications   Further airway obstruction from closing the mouth or pushing on the soft tissues under the chin.

Equipment

> Gloves

Psychosocial Considerations   This procedure is performed on the child with an altered level of consciousness. Speak to the child in a calm and soothing voice, as if he or she were fully conscious. Keep the family apprised of the

Table 4.2. Nursing Responsibilities

NURSING ACTIONS	RATIONALE
1. Determine that the child is unresponsive; don gloves.	Minimizes the potential damage from unnecessary resuscitation efforts.
2. Place the child in a supine position, turning the child as a unit (head, neck, and spine simultaneously.)	Minimizes the possibility of cervical spine injury, the potential for which exists in the unconscious child.
3. Place the fingers of one hand (not the thumb) under the bony part of the lower jaw at the chin and lift the chin upward. Place the other hand on the forehead.	Prevents obstruction; in unconscious children, upper airway obstruction is frequently the result of loss of tone in the submandibular muscles, which provide both direct support of the tongue and indirect support of the epiglottis.[2,6] The chin-lift method displaces the mandible anteriorly, thereby preventing the tongue from occluding the posterior pharynx.
4. Place a small towel roll under the child's neck and upper back, to maintain head position.	The relatively large size of the child's occiput creates a space at the nape of the neck, which must be maintained for proper positioning.
5. Reevaluate the airway status and respiratory effort; continue other airway support measures, if needed.	Determines whether further interventions are needed and subsequently initiated.
6. Document the child's response to the maneuver.	Communicates nursing interventions and observations to health-care professionals.

child's treatment; if they choose to remain in the room, have a support person stay with them to tend to their needs.

Nursing responsibilities are described in Table 4.3.

Jaw Thrust

Indications   The jaw thrust is a safe maneuver to open the airway when the potential for a cervical spine injury exists or in the unconscious child.

Contraindications   None.

Complications   None.

Equipment

Gloves

Psychosocial Considerations   This procedure is performed on the child with an altered level of consciousness. Speak to the child in a calm and soothing voice, as if she or he were fully conscious. Keep the family apprised of the child's treatment; if they choose to remain in the room, have a support person stay with them to tend to their needs.

Nursing responsibilities are described in Table 4.4.

Table 4.3. Nursing Responsibilities

NURSING ACTIONS	RATIONALE
1. Determine that the child is unresponsive.	Minimizes the potential damage from unnecessary resuscitation efforts.
2. Place the child in a supine position turning the child as a unit (head, neck and spine simultaneously).	Minimizes the possibility of a cervical spine injury, the potential for which exists in the unconscious child.
3. Gently lift the child's chin upward with the fingers of one hand while pushing down on the forehead with the other, tilting the head back slightly. In the infant, the head is placed in the neutral or sniffing position.	Slight extension of the head at the atlanto-occipital joint and forward displacement of the mandible can relieve an airway obstruction. This maneuver is also helpful in diverting inspired air away from the esophagus and into the trachea, as hyperextension of the head compresses the esophagus between the trachea and anterior portion of the cervical vertebrae.
4. Reevaluate the airway status and respiratory effort; continue other airway support measures, if needed.	Determines whether further interventions are needed and subsequently initiated.
5. Document the child's response to the maneuver.	Communicates nursing interventions and observations to health-care professionals.

Table 4.4. Nursing Responsibilities

NURSING ACTIONS	RATIONALE
1. Determine that the child is unresponsive.	Minimizes the risk of potential damage from unnecessary resuscitation efforts.
2. Place the child in a supine position, turning the child as a unit (head, neck, and spine simultaneously).	Minimizes the possibility of a cervical spine injury, the potential for which exists in the unconscious child.
3. Place two or three fingers under each side of the lower jaw at its angle and lift the jaw upward, maintaining this hold.[5]	As with the chin lift, the jaw-thrust maneuver displaces the mandible anteriorly, thereby preventing the tongue from occluding the posterior pharynx.
4. Reevaluate the airway status and respiratory effort; continue with other airway support measures, if needed.	Determines whether further interventions are needed and are subsequently initiated.
5. Document the child's response to the maneuver.	Communicates nursing interventions and observations to health-care professionals.

RELIEVING AN AIRWAY OBSTRUCTION

Indications   Complete airway obstruction, an ineffective cough and/or increased respiratory difficulty, accompanied by stridor.[5,6]

Contraindications   The infant and/or child who is able to cough, cry, or talk.

Complications   The potential for intra-abdominal injury is greater in infants; thus, a combination of back blows and chest thrusts is recommended.[5,6]

Equipment

> Gloves
> Pocket-type face mask

Psychosocial Considerations   During the procedure, explain to the child and family what is happening and why. After the procedure, explain to the child what has been done and why, if the child should ask. The child may have some abdominal discomfort afterward and will not understand why.

The family will need emotional support; they may have been trying to relieve the obstruction on the way into the emergency department and were not successful. Initiate interventions with appropriate support personnel.

Nursing responsibilities are described in Table 4.5.

Table 4.5.   Nursing Responsibilities for an Infant, a Conscious Child, or an Unconscious Child

INFANTS (LESS THAN 12 MONTHS OF AGE)	
NURSING ACTIONS	RATIONALE
1. Identify complete airway obstruction.	If the infant is able to cry or cough, the obstruction is not complete, and any interference could worsen the situation. If the infant is unable to cry, the obstruction could be complete.
2. Attempt to open the airway, using the head-tilt or chin-lift method. Lean forward, placing your cheek over the child's mouth and nose. Look, listen, and feel for breathing. Give two rescue breaths, 1–1$^{1}/_{2}$ seconds each, with enough force to see the chest rise and fall. If unsuccessful, reposition the child's head, and repeat the rescue breaths using the head tilt, chin lift, or jaw thrust maneuvers.	Basic procedures to open the airway are done to initiate breathing.
3. In the infant (less than 12 months of age), support the infant's head and neck with one hand firmly holding the jaw. With your forearm supported on your thigh, straddle the infant face down, head dependent.	Allows for secure positioning of the child.

Table 4.5.   *(cont.)*

INFANTS (LESS THAN 12 MONTHS OF AGE)	
NURSING ACTIONS	RATIONALE
4. With the heel of your other hand, deliver four back blows forcefully between the shoulder blades.[6] (See Figure 4.1.) Supporting the infant's head, sandwich the infant between your hands/arms, and turn the infant onto his or her back, head dependent.[6] Observe for any foreign body in the mouth.	Back blows may increase intrathoracic pressure and loosen the object. The infant's head is disproportionately large and is firmly supported to avoid injury.

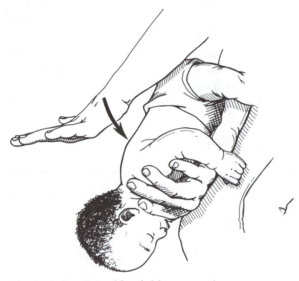

Figure 4.1.   Use of back blows to relieve an airway obstruction in an infant.

Table 4.5.   (*cont.*)

INFANTS (LESS THAN 12 MONTHS OF AGE)	
NURSING ACTIONS	RATIONALE
5. Place two fingers approximately one fingerwidth below the intermammary (nipple) line, above the xiphoid process. Deliver four chest thrusts at a depth of 0.5–1.0 inch (see Figure 4.2). Observe for any foreign bodies in the mouth.	Such thrusts increase intrathoracic pressure and force the residual volume in the lungs upward with enough pressure to expel the foreign body.

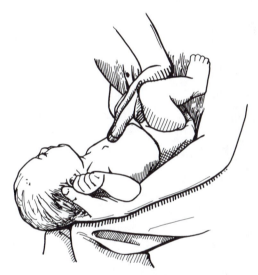

Figure 4.2.   Delivering chest thrusts to relieve an airway obstruction.

6. Repeat the sequence of back blows, chest thrusts, foreign body check, opening the airway, and attempting rescue breathing until the object is dislodged. Never perform a blind finger sweep; remove a foreign body only if it is visualized after using a chin lift or a jaw thrust.	As the infant becomes deprived of oxygen, the muscles relax, and maneuvers that were previously ineffective may become effective.

CONSCIOUS CHILD (1–8 YEARS OLD)	
NURSING ACTIONS	RATIONALE
1. See Step 1 for infant.	If the child is conscious, he or she may be using the "universal distress signal" of choking.
2. See Step 2 for infant.	
3. Stand behind the child, and wrap your arms around the child's waist.[6] Grasp one of your fists with your other hand. Place the thumb side of your fist in the child's midline	Hand placement at the xiphoid process or at the lower margin of the rib cage can result in damage to the internal organs.[6]

Table 4.5. (*cont.*)

CONSCIOUS CHILD (1–8 YEARS OLD)	
NURSING ACTIONS	RATIONALE

slightly above the navel and below
the rib cage.[6] (See Figure 4.3.)

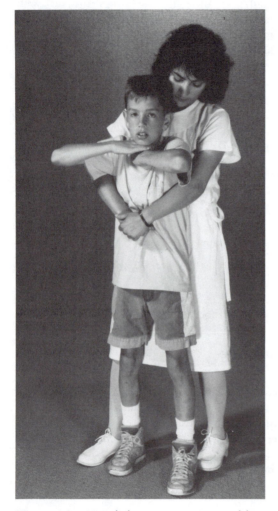

Figure 4.3.   Heimlich maneuver in an older,
awake child.

4. Press your fist into the child's abdomen with quick inward and upward thrusts. Deliver each thrust decisively. Six to ten thrusts can be delivered in succession.	Such thrusts increase intrathoracic pressure and force the residual volume in the lungs upward with enough pressure to expel the foreign body.
5. Check for a foreign body, and remove it with your index finger, with a sweeping action, only if visualized.	Remove object only if seen. Blind finger sweeps may lodge the object more firmly.

Table 4.5.   (*cont.*)

CONSCIOUS CHILD (1–8 YEARS OLD)	
NURSING ACTIONS	RATIONALE
6. Repeat the cycle of abdominal thrusts, foreign-body checks, opening the airway, and attempting to ventilate until the object is ejected.[6]	As the child becomes deprived of oxygen, the muscles relax, and maneuvers that were previously ineffective may become effective.[6]

UNCONSCIOUS CHILD (1–8 YEARS OLD)	
NURSING ACTIONS	RATIONALE
1. See Step 1 for infants.	
2. See Step 2 for infants.	
3. Kneel at the child's feet, or kneel astride the child's thighs. If the child is on a table or stretcher, stand at the child's feet. Place the heel of one hand on the abdominal midline slightly above the navel but well below the xiphoid process. Place the second hand directly on top of the first.[6]	Hand placement at the xiphoid process or the lower margin of the rib cage can result in damage to the internal organs.[6]
4. Press into the child's abdomen with quick inward and upward thrusts. Deliver each thrust decisively. Six to ten thrusts can be delivered in succession.[6]	Such thrusts increase intrathoracic pressure and force the residual volume in the lungs upward with enough pressure to expel the foreign body.
5. Check for a foreign body, and remove it with your index finger, with a sweeping action, only if visualized.	Remove object only if seen. Blind finger sweeps may lodge object more firmly.
6. Repeat the cycle of abdominal thrusts, foreign-body checks, opening the airway, and attempting to ventilate until the object is dislodged.[6]	As the child becomes deprived of oxygen, the muscles relax, and maneuvers that were previously ineffective may become effective.[6]
7. Document the child's response to relieving the airway obstruction and what type of object was retrieved (if applicable).	Communicates nursing interventions and observations to health-care professionals.

USING AIRWAY ADJUNCTS

Insertion of an Oropharyngeal Airway

Indications   An oropharyngeal airway is used to maintain airway patency in an unconscious infant or child. This airway adjunct, usually made of plastic, with a curved body and a short bite block, is designed to prevent the tongue from falling against the posterior pharyngeal wall, thereby maintaining an open airway. Most oropharyngeal airways are shaped to provide an air passage, as well as a route for oral suctioning.

Contraindications   Conscious infant or child.

Complications   Trauma to the tongue, mucous membranes, or gums, and bleeding. Pressure ulcerations can also result from improper positioning.[7] Gagging and vomiting in the conscious child.

Equipment

>   Tongue depressor
>   Suction device
>   Suction catheters (5 French to 14 French)
>   Oropharyngeal airways (all sizes)
>   Gloves, goggles, mask

Psychosocial Considerations   This procedure is performed on the child with an altered level of consciousness. Speak to the child in a calm and soothing voice, as if he or she were fully conscious. Keep the family apprised of the child's treatment; if they choose to remain in the room, have a support person stay with them to tend to their needs.
    Nursing responsibilities are described in Table 4.6.

INSERTION OF A NASOPHARYNGEAL AIRWAY

Indications   A nasopharyngeal airway is a soft rubber or plastic tube that provides a channel for the flow of oxygen into the posterior pharynx behind the tongue. This type of airway provides airway maintenance and is tolerated fairly well in the conscious child.

Contraindications   Severe facial, head, or nasal trauma.

Complications   Lacerations to the adenoidal tissue and nasal mucosa can result in bleeding and further airway obstruction.

Equipment

>   Suction device
>   Suction catheters (all sizes)
>   Nasal airways (12–36 French)
>   Water-soluble lubricant
>   Gloves, goggles, mask if needed

Psychosocial Considerations   This procedure is performed on the child with an altered level of consciousness. Speak to the child in a calm and soothing voice, as if he or she were fully conscious. Keep the family apprised of the child's treatment; if they choose to remain in the room, have a support person stay with them to tend to their needs.
    Nursing responsibilities are described in Table 4.7.

Table 4.6. Nursing Responsibilities

NURSING ACTIONS	RATIONALE
1. Establish that the child is unconscious.	An oral airway that is placed in an awake patient can stimulate vomiting and laryngospasm.[2]
2. Maintain a neutral head position.	Prevents airway obstruction.
3. Measure for the correct size of oral airway. Proper size is estimated by placing the airway next to the face, with the flange at the level of the central incisors and the bite block parallel to the hard palate.[2,5] The tip of an appropriately sized airway should reach the angle of the jaw.[2,5] (See Figure 4.4.)	An airway that is too small will push the tongue against the posterior pharynx,[5,7] obstructing the airway; an airway that is too large can obstruct the larynx.[5]

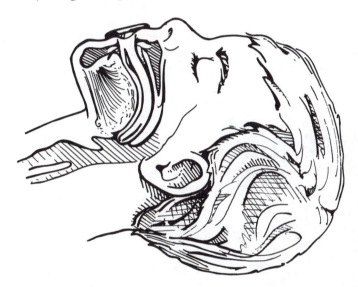

Figure 4.4. Correct placement of an oropharyngeal airway. The oropharyngeal airway is measured from the corner of the mouth to the angle of the jaw.

4. Insert a tongue depressor into the child's oropharynx, holding the tongue against the floor of the mouth. Position the oral airway over the tongue depressor and into the oropharynx.	Use of the tongue blade to position an oral airway is one of the safest methods, as it minimizes damage to the mucous membranes. An alternative method, placing an inverted airway into the mouth and rotating it into position as it reaches the back of the oropharynx, can result in damage to the mucous membranes, bleeding, and damage to the teeth.[13]
5. Reevaluate the airway status, and observe for complications.	

Table 4.6. (*cont.*)

NURSING ACTIONS	RATIONALE
6. Explain to the family the presence and function of the oropharyngeal airway.	Assists them in understanding their child's treatment.
7. Document the size of the airway used and the child's response to the procedure.	Communicates nursing interventions and observations to health-care professionals.

Table 4.7. Nursing Responsibilities

NURSING ACTIONS	RATIONALE
1. Establish that the child is unconscious or is conscious, but requires airway maintenance.	
2. Measure for correct size of nasal airway. Proper size is estimated by measuring the distance from the tip of the nose to the tragus of the ear (see Figure 4.5).[2,5]	An incorrect size of airway may injure nasopharyngeal tissues.

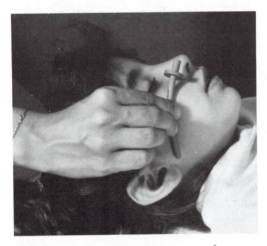

Figure 4.5.   Correct measurement of a nasopharyngeal airway.

3. Lubricate the airway, and insert it gently through the right nostril in a posterior direction, perpendicular to the facial plane; the bevel goes toward the nasal septum.[5]	Maintains airway patency.
4. Reevaluate the airway status and observe for complications.	Nasal airways are very compliant and can be easily obstructed by blood, mucus, or vomitus; thus, they may not be reliable.

Table 4.7.   (*cont.*)

NURSING ACTIONS	RATIONALE
5. Explain to the family the presence and function of the nasopharyngeal airway.	Assists them in understanding their child's treatment.
6. Document the size of the nasal airway used and the child's response to the procedure.	Communicates nursing interventions and observations to health-care professionals.

TRACHEAL INTUBATION

Though tracheal intubation was once performed primarily by an anesthesiologist or an otolaryngologist, it is now routinely performed by physicians, paramedics, nurse anesthetists, and transport nurses. Placement of a tube directly into the trachea offers several advantages, including the following:[2,5]

1. Maximizing oxygenation through the delivery of 100 percent oxygen.
2. Removal of carbon dioxide through hyperventilation.
3. Preventing gastric distention by isolating the trachea from the pharynx.
4. Allowing for the removal of blood, mucus, or meconium from the trachea by direct suctioning.
5. Providing a route of administration for several advanced life-support medications. (Atropine, Epinephrine and Lidocaine)
6. Permitting the application of positive end-expiratory pressure (PEEP).

In the trauma patient, aggressive airway management is critical. Airway compromise is the most life-threatening aspect of trauma in children, and the ability to control the airway often determines the success of resuscitation.[10] The use of endotracheal intubation is advocated with any of the following pediatric trauma scenarios:

1. A decreased level of consciousness (infant or child not responding appropriately to verbal stimuli)[9] or Glasgow Coma Scale score ≤ 7
2. Severe facial, neck, or chest injuries[9]
3. Systolic blood pressure of 20 mm Hg below the expected level[9]
4. A PaO_2 of 80 or less on supplemental oxygen[9]

Although infrequently performed, nasotracheal intubation offers several advantages over oral endotracheal intubation, including[8] (a) greater comfort than with the oral route, (b) less difficulty in securing the tube, (c) less chance of tube kinking and no chance of tube biting by the child, and (d) minimal movement with swallowing.

Nasotracheal intubation is technically a more difficult procedure and usually requires the assistance of a second health professional. In general, blind endotracheal intubation of children below the age of 6–8 years is more difficult, due to the anteriorly placed glottis. The technique is rarely addressed in the pediatric literature.

Oral Endotracheal Intubation

Indications   Endotracheal intubation is the most effective means of maintaining a patent airway for a prolonged period of time when the need for respiratory assistance will not resolve within minutes. It is used when rapid access to the airway is needed.

Contraindications An effective, short-term airway can be maintained through a basic maneuver; proficient personnel are not available to perform the procedure; or a complete airway obstruction exists, where a foreign body is not retrievable with forceps.

Complications Trauma to the teeth, gums, or tongue from instrumentation; expulsion, displacement, or obstruction of the tube; infection; laryngeal or tracheal edema; laryngospasm; right mainstream bronchus intubation.[2,8]

Equipment

> Laryngoscope (with extra batteries and bulbs)
> Blades
>> Straight blade (infants and young children)
>> Curved blade (older children and adolescents)
> Uncuffed tubes (infants to 8 years)
> Cuffed tubes (8 years and older)
> Stylet or ice
> Suction device
> Suction catheters (all sizes)
> Cardiac monitor/electrodes
> Gloves, goggles, mask
> Bag-valve-mask device
> Oxygen source
> Paralyzation and sedation medications, as ordered by the physician
> Soft restraints
> End tidal CO_2 detector
> Pulse oximeter

Psychosocial Considerations This procedure involves the face and mouth, which are highly sensitive and meaningful areas to the young child. Sedation must always accompany paralyzation with intubation. Assure the child that she or he will be able to breathe; explain why the child is unable to talk (e.g., "You have a tube in your throat to help you to breathe"). Encourage the child to communicate through eye blinking, finger movement, hand squeezes, and so forth.

The family must be prepared for what their child will look like with the endotracheal tube secured and connected to a ventilator or bag valve device. Encourage the family to touch and to talk to the child. Reassure them that the endotracheal tube is not permanent, that it is not painful to the child, and that the child has had medication that makes him or her sleepy and unable to move. Parents may become afraid when hearing the word "paralyzed" and may need a simple explanation that the child's inability to move is from medication and is not permanent.

Nursing responsibilities are described in Table 4.8.

Table 4.8. Nursing Responsibilities

NURSING ACTIONS	RATIONALE
1. Obtain the necessary equipment and ensure its working order; place the child on a cardiac monitor and pulse oximeter. Explain to the child (awake or unconscious), and the family, the need for the procedure, as time permits.	Endotracheal intubation cannot be performed unless the correct equipment is immediately available and in good working order; during intubation, bradycardia or other life-threatening dysrhythmias can occur.[5] An explanation prepares the child/family for the procedure. Time may not allow for this preparation.
2. Don gloves, goggles, and mask.	Complies with universal precautions.
3. Select correct size of laryngoscope blade and two endotracheal tubes. Tube size is estimated by the size of the outside diameter of the child's little finger or by this formula: age (in years) + 16, divided by 4.	The straight blade is recommended for infants because it provides better tongue displacement and better visualization of the relatively high and anterior larynx.[2,5] In children under the age of approximately 8 years, an uncuffed tube is recommended, as the normal subglottic narrowing provides for a snug fit; the cricoid cartilage then serves as a functional cuff. In children over the age of 8 years, a cuffed tube can be safely used. A rigid (or lighted)[12] stylet is sometimes fitted into the endotracheal tube, to maintain the desired curvature during insertion. Care must be taken to ensure that the distal end of the stylet is at least 2 cm proximal from the tip of the endotracheal tube, to minimize potential danger to the airway. If a stylet is not available, the tube can be placed in ice to increase its firmness.
4. Obtain and administer paralyzation and sedation medications, as ordered by the physician.	Facilitates tube placement.
5. Place the child's head in the sniffing (head-tilt) position. The child is supine, with the neck lifted slightly and the occiput flat on the surface. Gentle backward pressure is placed on the forehead, while directing the nares in a sniffing position. This position is contraindicated in the patient with a potential cervical spine injury.	Promote ease of direct visualization of vocal cords and surrounding structures.

Table 4.8. (*cont.*)

NURSING ACTIONS	RATIONALE
6. Hyperventilate the child with 100 percent oxygen using a bag-valve-mask device for several minutes prior to the intubation attempt.	Provides preoxygenation prior to brief disruption of ventilation for intubation.
7. Place the laryngoscope in your left hand, and open the child's mouth with your right hand. Note the time when the procedure is initiated.	Intubation attempts should not exceed 30 seconds.[5] If the child shows bradycardia (i.e., pulse < 80, infant; pulse < 60, child) or cyanosis, the procedure should be aborted and the child vigorously hyperventilated with 100 percent oxygen. Longer attempts will produce profound hypoxemia.[2,5]
8. Introduce the laryngoscope into the right side of the mouth, and sweep the tongue over to the left side; have suction readily available.	Allows for a channel in the right third of the mouth where the endotracheal tube is inserted.
9. If a curved blade is used, advance it gently until the tip is in the vallecula; if a straight blade is being used, the tip should be placed just under the epiglottis. Blade traction is exerted in an upward fashion in the direction of the long axis of the handle. It is important to not use the handle in a prying motion or as a fulcrum.	Displaces the base of the tongue and epiglottis anteriorly, exposing the vocal cords.
10. Once the vocal cords are visualized, the endotracheal tube is inserted until the black marker is at the level of the vocal cords. If the vocal cords are not easily visualized, slight external cricoid pressure may be helpful.	External cricoid pressure (Selleck maneuver) also avoids gastric inflation.[5]
11. Confirm correct tube placement. a. Auscultate breath sounds bilaterally at the apices and midaxillary lines, at the epigastrum, and at the sternal notch.	Definitive confirmation of correct tube placement by auscultation is difficult because breath sounds can be transmitted from the lungs to the abdomen when the tube is in the larynx. Conversely, sounds from the abdomen to the thorax can be transmitted when the tube is in the esophagus.[11] If unsure of tube placement, direct visualization of the tube through the vocal cords will verify placement.
b. Observe bilateral in the endotracheal tube.	Suggests correct placement because of the presence of moisture in the lungs.

Table 4.8. (*cont.*)

NURSING ACTIONS	RATIONALE
c. Observe symmetrical chest wall movement.	Chest expansion on only one side may indicate that the tube is in the corresponding mainstem bronchus and should be repositioned by withdrawing it slightly until both sides move equally.
d. Attach an end-tidal CO_2 detector between the big-valve device and the endotracheal tube.	A yellow color observed upon exhalation indicates correct placement.
12. Apply benzoin to the upper lip. Tape/tie the tube where the upper central incisors touch the endotracheal tube (see Figure 4.6).	Prevents dislodgment of the tube.

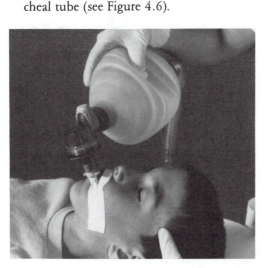

Figure 4.6. Endotracheal tube taped in place. The tube should not rest against the corner of the mouth. Note that the pop-off valve on the bag-valve device is occluded.

13. Obtain a chest x-ray to confirm the tube's placement (when time permits).	Radiographic assessment of the tube position should reveal the tube to be above the carina, in the mid third of the trachea, at the level of the second thoracic vertebrae.
14. Restrain the child appropriately.	Tube displacement is easily accomplished; thus, soft wrist and ankle restraints are recommended.
15. Reevaluate tube placement at frequent intervals and observe for complications.	
16. Explain to the family and the child why the tube is in place, how it	Assists in their understanding of the procedure.

Table 4.8. (*cont.*)

NURSING ACTIONS	RATIONALE
works, why the child cannot speak, and so forth.	
17. Document the time of intubation, the size of the endotracheal tube, confirmation of the placement, medications administered, how the child tolerated the procedure, and changes in the child's condition.	Communicates nursing interventions and observations to health-care professionals.

ASSISTING WITH NEEDLE CRICOTHYROTOMY

Indications   A needle cricothyrotomy is indicated for short-term airway support when all other nonsurgical attempts at ventilation have failed, with complete airway obstruction, not relieved with the Heimlich maneuver, and in severe maxillofacial trauma. The American College of Surgeons recommends this procedure on children 12 years of age and less,[13] although the age recommendations are controversial. A needle cricothyrotomy provides for minimal exchange of oxygen and carbon dioxide and thus is recommended only for brief periods of time (30 to 45 minutes).[13]

Contraindication   Airway obtainable through any other airway maneuver.

Complications   Bleeding at the site of needle insertion, esophageal perforation, and pneumothorax due to the high pressures required for ventilation. This technique does not allow for suctioning.

Equipment

> Large-bore intravenous over-the-needle-catheter needle (12-gauge or 14-gauge[13]; 14-gauge or 16-gauge[5])
> 3.0 endotracheal tube adapter (removed from the 3.0 endotracheal tube)
> 10-cc syringe
> Alcohol wipes
> Bag-valve device or jet insufflation device
> Oxygen source
> Cardiac monitor and electrodes
> Gloves, goggles, mask
> Benzoin or adhesive spray
> Tape
> Suture material

Psychosocial Considerations   Even though the child is unconscious, explain what is happening to her or him. The parents will need emotional support; see Chapter 2, Psychosocial Considerations for the Child and Family.
   Nursing responsibilities are described in Table 4.9.

Table 4.9.   Nursing Responsibilities

NURSING ACTION	RATIONALE
1. Obtain the necessary equipment and ensure its working order; place the child on a cardiac monitor. Explain to the child (awake or unconscious) and the family the need for the procedure, as time permits.	Assists with efficient performance of procedure. Assists in their understanding of the child's treatment.
2. Don gloves, goggles and mask.	Complies with universal precautions.
3. Place the child in the neutral position or with the neck slightly hyperextended.	The neutral position should be used if there is any possibility of a cervical spine injury; access to the neck is difficult, due to the child's small stature.
4. Identify the cricothyroid membrane. Place two fingers in the suprasternal notch, and palpate the trachea. Slowly palpate the trachea upward, toward the head, until the first cartilage ring is felt. This is the cricoid cartilage. The next ring palpated is the thyroid cartilage, and in between them lies the cricothyroid membrane (see Figure 4.7).	In adult males, the cricothyroid membrane lies directly below the Adam's apple. In women and children, however, the thyroid cartilage is not as prominent.

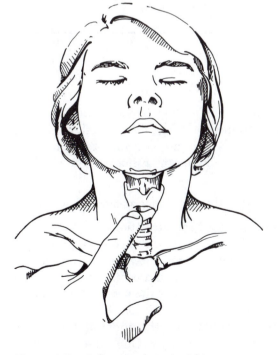

Figure 4.7.   Palpating the cricoid in preparation for cricothyroidotomy.

Table 4.9.   (*cont.*)

NURSING ACTION	RATIONALE
5. Attach the catheter-over-the-needle device to the 10-cc syringe. Cleanse the skin with the alcohol wipes.	
6. Directing the catheter at a 45-degree angle caudally, pierce the skin at the mid cricothyroid membrane.	Allows for entry into the trachea.
7. Aspirate continuously after piercing the skin.	Aspiration of a free flow of air signals entry into the trachea.
8. Advance the catheter, remove the needle, and attach the catheter to either the 3.0 endotracheal adapter and either a bag-valve device or a jet insufflation device.	Allows for inflation of the lungs. The bag-valve device, without a pop-off valve, can be used in conjunction with the catheter-over-the-needle device and a 3.0 endotracheal tube adapter.
9. Evaluate breath sounds while oxygenating the child.	Air exchange with this procedure is poor and limited to a brief period of time. Hypercapnea is a serious problem and can be hazardous in the child with a head injury.
10. Explain to the family the equipment being used.	Assists in their understanding of the child's treatment.
11. Document the size of needle inserted, the type of oxygenation device used, and any changes in the child's condition.	Communicates nursing interventions and observations to health-care professionals.

ASSISTING WITH SURGICAL CRICOTHYROTOMY

Indications   A surgical cricothyrotomy is indicated when an acute upper airway obstruction exists, endotracheal intubation fails, and ventilation is inadequate or impossible. Age recommendations are controversial, but it is generally recommended that surgical cricothyrotomy is not done in children less than 12 years of age.[13]

Contraindication   Airway maintainable through other airway measures.

Complications   Similar to those of endotracheal intubation but also include laceration of the cricothyroid artery, false passage of the endotracheal tube, right mainstem intubation, esophageal perforation, and subcutaneous or mediastinal emphysema.[2,11] A surgical cricothyrotomy is a potentially dangerous procedure in children because the cricoid cartilage is the narrowest portion of the airway in a child less than 8 years of age. In addition, laceration of the cricothyroid artery, which extends horizontally over the upper portion of the cricoid membrane, can result in extensive bleeding.[11] One common error is inserting the endotracheal tube too far and entering the right mainstem bronchus. If a cuffed tube is used, the tube should not be advanced once the cuff has entered the membrane.

Equipment

Appropriate size of endotracheal tube
Scalpel with #11 blade
Alcohol wipes
Bag-valve device without pop-off valve
Oxygen source
Suction device
Suction catheters (all sizes)
Cardiac monitor/electrodes
Gloves, goggles, mask
Benzoin/adhesive spray
Tape or suture material

Psychosocial Considerations Even though the child is unconscious, explain what is happening to her or him. The parents will need emotional support; see Chapter 2, Psychosocial Considerations for the Child and Family.

Nursing responsibilities are described in Table 4.10.

Table 4.10. Nursing Responsibilities

NURSING ACTION	RATIONALE
1. Obtain the necessary equipment and ensure its working order; place the child on a cardiac monitor; explain to the child (awake or unconscious), and the family, the need for the procedure, as time permits.	Assists with efficient performance of the procedure. Assists in the family's understanding of the child's treatment.
2. Don gloves, goggles and mask.	Complies with universal precautions.
3. Place the child in the neutral position or with the neck slightly hyperextended.	The neutral position should be used if there is any possibility of a cervical spine injury. Slight hyperextension may allow for better access to the neck, which is difficult due to the child's small stature.
4. Assist with cleansing the area.	
5. The physician makes a small (1.0 to 1.5 cm) horizontal incision with the scalpel at the level of the cricothyroid membrane. The skin is incised and the membrane located. A second incision can then be made directly through the membrane. An alternative approach is to enter the skin and membrane during the initial incision.	
6. The physician inserts the endotracheal tube and directs it caudally through the membrane.	
7. Evaluate breath sounds while oxygenating the child with the bag-valve device.	Assures correct placement of the tube.

Table 4.10.   (*cont.*)

NURSING ACTION	RATIONALE
8. Secure the endotracheal tube by using benzoin or an adhesive spray, as well as waterproof tape, or by suturing the tube in place.	
9. Explain to the family the equipment being used.	Assists in their understanding of the child's treatment.
10. Document the size of the endotracheal tube, the oxygenation device used, and any changes in the child's condition.	Communicates nursing interventions and observations to health-care professionals.

SUCTIONING

Suctioning is employed to clear the mouth, pharynx and trachea of secretions, blood, vomitus, or meconium; suctioning is also done to stimulate a productive cough. Suctioning devices are powered by batteries, wall current, or a hand-powered vacuum. Most suction catheters have a proximally located side opening, or port, which controls the amount of negative pressure. Suctioning is performed with a tonsillar-tip (Yankauer) or flexible plastic catheter.

Oropharyngeal and Posterior Pharyngeal Suctioning

Indications   Oropharyngeal and posterior pharyngeal suctioning are performed in the presence of secretions, blood, vomitus, or meconium. Suctioning can also be done to stimulate a productive cough. Noisy respirations, tachycardia, tachypnea, and restlessness may indicate the need for suctioning. Cyanosis is a *late* sign of hypoxia.

Contraindications   Epiglottitis, due to the potential for laryngospasm and respiratory arrest.

Complications   Trauma to the mucous membranes and bradycardia.

Equipment

> Tonsillar-tip catheter
> Suction catheters (all sizes),[5]
>   neonate 8 French
>   6 month 8–10 French
>   1–2 years 10 French
>   5 years 14 French
>   8–10 years 14 French
> Suction tubing
> Suction device
> Irrigating solution
> Gloves, goggles, mask

Psychosocial Considerations   The child, already in distress, may be frightened by the noise of the suction device. Reassurance and a calm manner help the child to cope with the procedure.

Nursing responsibilities are described in Table 4.11.

Table 4.11. Nursing Responsibilities

NURSING ACTIONS	RATIONALE
1. Explain to the child and the family the need for suctioning.	Enhances their understanding and cooperation.
2. Connect the suction catheter to the tubing of the suction device.	
3. Wash your hands; don gloves, goggles and mask.	Complies with universal precautions.
4. Gently open the child's mouth and insert the catheter without suction applied. Do not insert the catheter into the posterior pharynx in the conscious child. Large particles may be effectively removed with the suction tubing only.	Care must be taken when inserting the catheter in the posterior pharynx, as this may stimulate a vagal response, resulting in bradycardia. In the conscious child, insertion of the catheter into the posterior pharynx may also elicit a gag response.
5. Turn on the suction to the desired negative pressure. Apply suction by occluding the on/off port.	
6. Repeat as needed after cleaning the catheter with irrigating solution.	
7. Inspect the oropharynx for further secretions.	
8. Document the child's response to the suctioning; type, amount, and odor of suctioned material; changes in heart or respiratory rates; and duration of suctioning.	Communicates nursing interventions and observations to health-care professionals.

Nasopharyngeal Suctioning

Indications   Nasopharyngeal suctioning is used to remove blood and/or secretions from the nasal passages and posterior pharynx in the conscious or unconscious child. Noisy respirations, tachycardia, tachypnea, and restlessness may indicate the need for suctioning.

Contraindications   Head injury with suspected basilar skull fracture; maxillofacial trauma.

Complications   Trauma to the nasal mucous membranes and bleeding.

Equipment

> Suction catheters (all sizes) (refer to p. 56 for sizes)
> Suction tubing
> Suction unit
> Irrigating solution
> Sterile gloves; goggles; mask
> Water-soluble lubricant

Psychosocial Considerations   The child may feel uncomfortable during the procedure. The young child may have fears about where the catheter is going in his or her body. Speaking calmly and offering reassurance helps the child during the procedure.

Nursing responsibilities are described in Table 4.12.

Endotracheal Suctioning

Indications   Endotracheal suctioning is performed to remove blood and/or secretions from the endotracheal tube. It is a sterile procedure. Noisy respirations, tachycardia, tachypnea, restlessness, or poor arterial blood gases may indicate the need for suctioning.

Contraindications   Increased intracranial pressure; however, the situation must be individualized as to the risk of hypoxia versus increased intracranial pressure during suctioning.

Complications   Hypoxia, trauma to the tracheal bronchial mucosa, cardiac dysrhythmias, and increased intracranial pressure.

Table 4.12. Nursing Responsibilities

NURSING ACTIONS	RATIONALE
1. Explain to the child and the family the need for suctioning, as time permits.	Enhances their understanding and cooperation. Time may not permit this preparation.
2. Wash your hands; put on gloves, goggles and mask.	Complies with universal precautions.
3. Connect the suction catheter to the tubing of the suction device.	
4. Measure for the correct size of catheter. Length can be measured from the nares to the lobe of the ear and then to the thyroid cartilage, just above the cricoid membrane.	Assures correct length of catheter for insertion.
5. Lubricate the catheter, and gently insert it into the nostril and posterior pharynx.	Reduces trauma to the nasal passages.
6. Turn on the suction device to the desired negative pressure. Apply suction by occluding the on/off port, and gently withdraw catheter. Suctioning should be limited to 5 seconds and 80 to 120 mm Hg of negative pressure.	Decreases risk of hypoxemia and mucosal trauma.
7. Repeat, as needed, after cleaning the catheter with irrigating solution.	
8. Document the child's response to the suctioning, the type, amount and odor of suctioned material, changes in heart or respiratory rates, and duration of suctioning.	Communicates nursing interventions and observations to health-care professionals.

Equipment

Suction catheters (all sizes) (refer to p. 56 for sizes)
Suction tubing
Suction device
Sterile irrigating solution
Sterile gloves, goggles, mask
Water-soluble lubricant
Oxygen source
Bag-valve device

Psychosocial Considerations   The child requiring endotracheal suctioning may still be capable of auditory and tactile perceptions even though he or she may have received sedation and a paralytic agent. The intubated child requires age-appropriate explanations of the procedure prior to its performance, including any sensations that she or he may experience.

Nursing responsibilities are described in Table 4.13.

Table 4.13. Nursing Responsibilities

NURSING ACTIONS	RATIONALE
1. Explain to the child and the family the need for endotracheal suctioning, as time permits.	Enhances their understanding and cooperation. Time may not allow for this preparation.
2. Note the child's cardiac monitor and pulse oximetry readings.	Endotracheal suctioning can result in hypoxia and/or bradycardia, due to vagal stimulation; thus, close monitoring of the vital signs is important.
3. Wash your hands; don gloves, goggles and mask.	Complies with universal precautions.
4. Connect the suction catheter to the tubing of the suction device and set the suction pressures between 80 and 120 mm Hg of negative pressure.	A limit of 80–120 mm Hg decreases the chance of mucosal damage.
5. Ventilate the child with 100% oxygen for several minutes. Auscultate anterior lungs bilaterally.	Ensures that the child is well oxygenated. Auscultation provides data to evaluate the effectiveness of the procedure.
6. Lubricate the appropriate size of catheter with sterile water, and gently insert it into the endotracheal tube and advance it to the level of the carina, using strict aseptic technique.	Lubrication may minimize frictional resistance during insertion.
7. Apply suction by occluding the on/off port, and gently withdrawing the catheter with a twisting motion. Limit the procedure to 5 seconds.	Jabbing, uneven movements of the catheter will damage the tracheal mucosa. Even when done properly, there is some irritation of the tracheal mucosa.

Table 4.13.   *(cont.)*

NURSING ACTIONS	RATIONALE
8. Ventilate between attempts and after the procedure, with 100% oxygen.	Suctioning can result in hypoxia, thus, supplemental oxygenation following this procedure is imperative.
9. Return the child to the source of oxygenation, such as bag-valve device or ventilator. Auscultate anterior lungs bilaterally.	
10. Comfort the child during and after the procedure.	
11. Document the child's response to suctioning, the type and amount of suctioned secretions, any changes in heart rate and respiratory effort, and breath sounds both pre- and post-suctioning.	Communicates nursing interventions and observations to health-care professionals.

REPLACING A TRACHEOSTOMY TUBE

Indications   A tracheostomy tube may become occluded from secretions or mucus and may require immediate replacement[16] if suctioning does not relieve the obstruction. Accidental decannulation is another indication.[16] Indications of an airway obstruction include stridor, noisy respirations, tachycardia, tachypnea, unconsciousness, restlessness, or cyanosis (a late sign). Silent respiratory effort and no air movement indicate complete airway obstruction.

Contraindications   Patent airway.

Complications   Inability to insert tracheostomy tube may result in respiratory compromise. Improper placement outside the trachea can create a false channel that does not permit adequate air exchange.

Equipment

> New tracheostomy tube with ties in place
> Tracheostomy tube one size smaller than the previous tube
> Scissors
> Suction device
> Suction catheters (all sizes)
> Gauze
> Sterile saline irrigation
> Oxygen source
> Bag-valve device
> Sterile gloves, goggles, mask

Psychosocial Considerations   Removing the tracheostomy tube of the already frightened child in respiratory distress is certain to heighten her or his anxiety. Show the child the new tube, and assure the child that it will be replaced, to help him or her to breathe better. Allow the parent to participate if he or she feels comfortable in assisting.

Nursing responsibilities are described in Table 4.14.

Table 4.14. Nursing Responsibilities

NURSING ACTIONS	RATIONALE
1. Explain to the child and family the need to replace the tracheostomy tube, if time permits.	Enhances their understanding and cooperation. Time may not allow for this preparation.
2. Wash your hands, and don sterile gloves, goggles and the mask. Obtain the assistance of another individual (parent, or other health-care professional).	Prevents infective injury to patient and nurse; additional assistance may be required to help with positioning, suctioning, and so forth.
3. Remove a new tube from the box, with the obturator in place; keep it within reach.	
4. Ventilate the child with 100% oxygen.[14]	
5. Position the child with the neck hyperextended. A towel roll behind the shoulders may help with positioning. The second person helps to hold the child still.	Exposes the tracheostomy site and forces the trachea closer to the skin.
6. Cut the ties on the old tracheostomy tube while holding the tube in place.	A forceful cough can easily dislodge the tube if it is not held in place.
7. If time permits, lubricate the new tracheostomy tube by dipping it into normal saline solution. Following the downward curve, remove the old tracheostomy tube. While removing the old tube, keep your eyes on the stoma.	
8. Insert the new tube, following the curve, into the stoma. If the tube is difficult to insert, reposition the child's head, and repeat your attempt. Inserting the tube during inhalation may also be helpful. If this is still unsuccessful, try inserting the tube that is one size smaller. Artificial ventilation can be given through the stoma site if necessary, or the stoma site can be covered with a gloved finger, and ventilation (using a bag-valve mask device) can be used to provide oxygenation.[14]	
9. Remove the obturator and hold the tube firmly in place.	A cough can dislodge the new tube.
10. Securely fasten the ties around the child's neck with a triple knot. Only one fingertip should fit between the neck and the ties. Suction through the tracheostomy tube if necessary.	Prevents skin irritation.

Table 4.14.   (*cont.*)

NURSING ACTIONS	RATIONALE
11. Document the size of the tracheostomy tube removed and inserted, the condition of the stoma, the ease of insertion, whether suctioning was needed, and how the child tolerated the procedure.	Communicates nursing interventions and observations to health-care professionals.

REFERENCES

1. Orlowski JP. Pediatric cardiopulmonary resuscitation. Emerg Med Clin North Am 1983;1:3; 5.
2. Albarran-Sotelo R, et al. Textbook of advanced cardiac life support. 2nd ed. Dallas: American Heart Association, 1987; 257; 261; 28; 30; 32–33, 262; 34.
3. Holbrook PR. On opening the airway. Emerg Med 1982;14:152; 141.
4. Crowley CM, Morrow AI. A comprehensive approach to the child in respiratory failure. Crit Care Q 1980;3:33.
5. Chameides L, ed. Textbook of pediatric advanced life support. Dallas: American Academy of Pediatrics and American Heart Association, 1988;11; 16; 13; 17; 25; 28; 29; 34; 33; 26.
6. Albarran-Sotelo R, Flint LS, Kelly KJ, eds. Instructor's manual for basic life support. Dallas: American Heart Association, 1987;61; 68; 69; 70.
7. Escher-Neidig JR. Pediatric respiratory arrest: Emergency airway management in the critical care setting. Crit Care Nurse 1988;8:22; 28.
8. Hughes WT, Buescher ES. Pediatric procedures, 2nd ed. Philadelphia: W.B. Saunders, 1980;207; 222; 225.
9. Morse TS. The child with multiple injuries. Emerg Med Clin North Am 1983;1:177; 178.
10. Eichelberger MR. Life threatening episodes in infants and children: Trauma. Symposium on life threatening episodes—the infant/child difference. Kalamazoo, Michigan: Upjohn, 1983.
11. Silverman BK, ed. Advanced pediatric life support. Dallas: American Academy of Pediatrics and American College of Emergency Physicians, 1989;5; 6; 72; 73.
12. Stewart R. Field airway control for the trauma patient. In: Campbell J., ed. Basic trauma life support—advanced prehospital care. 2nd ed. New Jersey: Prentice-Hall, 1988;79; 83.
13. Advanced trauma life manual. 2nd ed. Chicago: Committee on Trauma, American College of Surgeons 1984;25; 26; 27.
14. Ruddy RM. Section editor. Illustrated techniques of pediatric emergency procedures. In: Fleisher G, Ludwig S, eds. Textbook of pediatric emergency medicine. 2nd ed. Baltimore: Williams & Wilkins, 1988;1291.

5

Procedures Involving the Respiratory System

Linda Karen Manley

OVERVIEW OF PEDIATRIC RESPIRATORY DIFFERENCES

Cardiopulmonary arrest in children is usually the end result of progressive respiratory or circulatory failure, both of which begin as clinically distinct syndromes.[1] *Hypoxemia,* resulting from apnea or inadequate alveolar ventilation, occurs more rapidly in children than in adults, due to their higher metabolic rate and increased oxygen consumption.

Respiratory failure is a clinical state characterized by inadequate elimination of carbon dioxide and/or inadequate oxygenation at the alveolar–capillary membrane.[1] This condition can be caused by airway disease, lung pathology, central nervous system depression (e.g., due to drugs or head trauma), or foreign body obstruction. Respiratory failure is often preceded by a compensated state, characterized by an increased work of breathing, in which the child can maintain adequate gas exchange.[1] Recognizing the subtle signs and symptoms of this compensated state is imperative for emergency nurses caring for pediatric patients. As respiratory failure progresses, the result is end-organ dysfunction due to tissue hypoxia and acidosis; death or anoxic brain damage quickly ensues.

Early recognition of the subtle signs and symptoms of respiratory distress should be in every nurse's repertoire of skills. A respiratory assessment is one of the most important components of the pediatric evaluation. First, the nurse determines the responsiveness of the infant or child. Gentle shaking of the infant or child should elicit a response. If the child is conscious but struggling to breathe, the nurse should place the child in the position of greatest comfort, usually with the head of the bed elevated.

Next, the nurse assesses the child's level of consciousness because early signs of hypoxia and respiratory failure include a change in the child's level of consciousness (i.e., agitation, restlessness, or irritability), progressing to lethargy and obtundation. Evaluating the infant's level of consciousness is more difficult but can be judged by muscle tone, strength of the cry, response to parents, and activity level. By 2 months of age, most infants can focus on their parents' faces. Failure of a child to recognize or respond to his or her parent may be an early sign of reduced cerebral perfusion.

The nurse then assesses the child's respiratory rate. Respiratory rates in children are age dependent (see Table 1.2 in the Physical Assessment and Triage chapter). Tachypnea may be the first sign of respiratory distress in infants. Quiet tachypnea, which is tachypnea without other signs of respiratory distress—such as retractions, grunting, flaring—commonly results from nonpulmonary diseases (e.g., diabetic ketoacidosis, poisonings, severe dehydration).[1] This type of tachypnea represents the body's attempt to maintain a normal pH by increasing minute ventilation and eliminating carbon dioxide. A slow respiratory rate in an acutely ill or injured child is an ominous sign, which may be caused by fatigue, hypothermia, or central nervous system depression.

The nurse observes the child's respiratory effort, such as substernal, suprasternal, and intercostal retractions, nasal flaring, head bobbing, and positioning (upright, leaning forward). Increased work of breathing results in a greater proportion of the cardiac output being delivered to the respiratory muscles and more carbon dioxide production. When the work of breathing exceeds the ability to adequately oxygenate the tissue, acidosis ensues.[1]

During normal respiration, the ribs and sternum support the lungs and help keep it expanded. The diaphragm, the main muscle of respiration in children, and the intercostal muscles generate negative intrathoracic pressure. Excessive negative intrathoracic pressure, coupled with a normally pliable rib cage, leads to retractions.

Stridor, a high-pitched inspiratory sound, is the hallmark of an upper airway obstruction, occurring between the supraglottic space and the lower trachea;[1] stridor can be caused by infection (croup or epiglottitis), a foreign body, or a congenital anomaly. *Grunting* occurs in diseases in which there is an accumulation of interstitial or alveolar fluid (e.g., pneumonia, congestive heart failure); grunting is produced by the premature closure of the glottis during early expiration and is accompanied by active chest wall contraction.[1] Grunting leads to increased airway pressure, which helps to preserve or increase the functional residual volume.

Cyanosis is a *late* and inconsistent sign of respiratory failure and is dependent on the hemoglobin concentration. For example, in hypovolemic shock, if the hemoglobin is less than 5.9 grams, cyanosis will not be noted despite the presence of severe hypoxia. Cyanosis is best observed in the oral mucous membranes and the nail beds. Bilateral auscultation of the chest may reveal either wheezing, indicating bronchial spasm or obstruction, or rales, suggesting the presence of alveolar fluid.

Finally, the nurse (a) reports any respiratory difficulty to the physician in charge, (b) initiates respiratory support measures if indicated, and (c) documents nursing observations and interventions.

APPLYING OXYGEN DELIVERY SYSTEMS

Oxygen delivery systems are divided into "low-flow" and "high-flow" systems.[2] A *low-flow system* is one in which the gas flow is insufficient to meet all inspiratory flow requirements, and thus, outside air is introduced into the system. Examples of low-flow systems are the nasal cannula and the simple oxygen mask. A *high-flow system* adds a reservoir and therefore is able to supply the total inspired flow rate required by the patient.[1] The nurse should obtain a verbal or written order for supplemental oxygen or should follow hospital protocol for administering oxygen in emergent situations. Oxygen is a drug and requires a physician's order.

Psychosocial Considerations

Children do not like having anything near their faces, and they are already fearful when having difficulty breathing; having a mask or cannula on their face could make them even more anxious. Children need a calm and reassuring explanation of what will happen and how it will feel (i.e., cool, moist air). Placing a mask by the cheek first or over the head may help the child to adjust better. Alternatively, less anxiety may occur if the oxygen device is placed prior to the flow of oxygen. With cool mist, children sometimes think that the mist is smoke from a fire; carefully explain what it is and its intended purpose. Praise the child for being cooperative.

The family may need assistance in helping their child to keep the oxygen device on and may need reassurance to better assist their child.

Nasal Cannula

The nasal cannula (n/c) is a low-flow oxygen delivery device consisting of two short plastic prongs arising from a circular tube, which delivers oxygen (O_2) through the nasal passages into the posterior pharynx.

Indications   The nasal cannula is indicated in infants or children who require only a modest ($\leq 30\%$) amount of supplemental oxygen.

Contraindications   Any child who requires a precise concentration of oxygen, high-flow oxygen (more than 6 L/min), or additional humidification.

Complications   Irritation and crusting of the nares and mucous membranes.

Equipment

> Infant nasal cannula
> Child nasal cannula
> Adult nasal cannula
> Humidified O_2 source
> $^1/_2''$ tape
> Water-soluble lubricant

Nursing responsibilities are described in Table 5.1.

Masks

Simple Face Mask

The simple face mask is a low-flow device that delivers between 35 and 60% oxygen with a flow rate of 6-10 L/min.[1] Oxygen enters the mask via plastic

Table 5.1.   Nursing Responsibilities

NURSING ACTIONS	RATIONALE
1. Explain to the child and the family the need for oxygen. For example, say, "This special air will help you breathe better."	Enhances their understanding and cooperation.
2. Enlarge the loop of the cannula so that it will easily slip over both of the child's ears. Then, place the prongs into the nares and tighten the loop. The loop should always remain in front and should not encircle the face. If the child is particularly active, place a small piece of ½" tape over the cannula on both sides of the face (see Figure 5.1). Also, the prongs can be cut to decrease irritation in a young infant.	When adjusting the loop, ensure that it is not too tight, as this may cause the prongs to slip out of position and may potentially damage the mucous membranes of the nose.[3] A water-soluble lubricant applied to the nares avoids nasal mucous membrane irritation with prolonged n/c use.

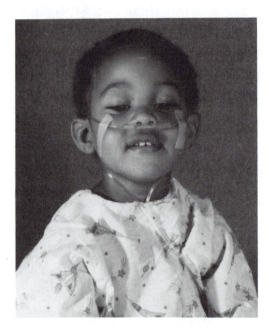

Figure 5.1.   Taping the nasal cannula to the cheeks of a young child assists in securing and hinders removal of the cannula.

3. Adjust the O$_2$ flow to the prescribed delivery rate.	
4. Document the method of oxygen delivery, the oxygen flow rate, and the patient's response to the therapy (respiratory effort, skin color, level of consciousness).	Communicates the nursing interventions and observations to health-care professionals.

tubing, and outside air enters through ports on the sides of the mask and between the mask and the face.[1]

Indications   The simple face mask is indicated in infants and children who require modestly enriched oxygen environments and who have good respiratory effort.

Contraindications   Need for a reliable, high (> 60%) concentration of oxygen.

Complications   None.

Equipment

> Appropriate size of mask: infant, pediatric, or adult size
> Humidified O_2 source

Nursing responsibilities are described in Table 5.2.

Venturi Mask
The Venturi principle is based on the premise that a stream ("jet") of 100% oxygen flowing rapidly through a narrow tube pulls in room air through side ports.[2] The size of the jet and side ports determines the proportions of air and oxygen. Thus, the Venturi mask is designed to deliver an exact oxygen concentration that is independent of the child's respiratory rate. Most Venturi masks can deliver 24, 28, 35, 40, or 50% oxygen.

Indications   The Venturi mask is indicated where there is a need for delivery of a specific concentration of O_2, up to 50%.

Contraindications   Any emergent condition in which the child requires a high percentage (> 60%) of supplemental oxygen.

Complications   None.

Equipment

> Venturi mask: pediatric or adult
> Humidified oxygen source

Nursing responsibilities are described in Table 5.3.

Partial and Full Nonrebreathing Masks
Partial and full nonrebreathing masks are simple face masks with an added reservoir bag. During exhalation, oxygen flows into the reservoir bag, together with the first third of the child's exhaled gases.[1] This portion of the exhaled gas remains in the upper airways and does not participate in respiratory gas exchange during the prior breath; thus, it is oxygen enriched.[1] Partial and full nonrebreathing masks are useful in providing oxygen concentrations of 50-60% at a flow rate of 10-12 L/min.[1] During inspiration, the child draws oxygen from the reservoir bag and, potentially, from the room via the side ports.[2,3]

There are two major differences between the partial and the full nonrebreathing mask. The full nonrebreathing mask has valves incorporated into the side ports to prevent the entry of room air during inspiration, plus an additional valve between the reservoir bag and mask to prevent gas flow back into the reservoir bag from the mask during exhalation.[1] The partial nonrebreathing mask has neither of these valves.[1]

Table 5.2.   Nursing Responsibilities

NURSING ACTIONS	RATIONALE
1. Explain to the child and the family the need for oxygen.	Enhances their understanding and cooperation.
2. Obtain an appropriate size of oxygen mask. The correct size is determined by a tight fit. The mask should extend from the bridge of the nose to the cleft of the chin. Attach the mask to a humidified oxygen source; adjust it to the desired flow rate, with a minimum oxygen flow of 6 L/min.	Humidified oxygen decreases irritation to the mucous membranes.
3. Place the mask over the child's face, starting from the nose downward, and adjust the nose clip and head strap. Methods to enhance oxygen delivery are by holding the O_2 over the child's head or by using blow-by O_2 (see Figure 5.2).	Too loose a fit will not ensure adequate oxygen delivery.

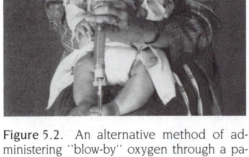

Figure 5.2.   An alternative method of administering "blow-by" oxygen through a paper cup attached to oxygen tubing.

4. Document the method of oxygen delivery, the oxygen flow rate, and the child's response to the therapy (respiratory effort, skin color, level of consciousness).	Communicates the nursing interventions and observations to health-care professionals.

Table 5.3. Nursing Responsibilities

NURSING ACTIONS	RATIONALE
1. Explain to the child and the family the need for oxygen.	Enhances their understanding and cooperation.
2. Obtain an appropriate size of Venturi mask, and attach it to the oxygen source; adjust it to the desired flow rate.	The Venturi mask is designed to deliver a preset amount of oxygen at a given flow rate.
3. Place the mask over the child's face, starting from the nose downward, and adjust the nose clip and head strap (as described in Table 5.3, regarding the nursing actions for the simple face mask).	Too loose a fit will not ensure adequate oxygen delivery.
4. Document the method of oxygen delivery, the O_2 flow rate, and the child's response to therapy (respiratory effort, skin color, level of consciousness).	Communicates the nursing interventions and observations to health-care professionals.

Indications   The partial and full nonrebreathing masks are indicated when there is a need for a high concentration of oxygen ($> 60\%$) in a child with adequate respiratory effort.

Contraindications   Apnea, poor respiratory effort.

Complications   None.

Equipment

> Partial and full nonrebreathing masks: pediatric or adult size
> Humidified oxygen source

Nursing responsibilities are described in Table 5.4.

Table 5.4. Nursing Responsibilities

NURSING ACTIONS	RATIONALE
1. Explain to the child and the family the need for oxygen.	Enhances their understanding and cooperation.
2. Obtain the appropriate size of oxygen mask. Attach the oxygen mask to the oxygen source, and fully inflate the reservoir bag. In general, a flow rate of greater than 12 L/min is required to inflate the attached oxygen reservoir bag. Adjust the oxygen flow into the mask to prevent reservoir bag collapse.[1]	Allows for proper delivery of oxygen.
3. Place the mask over the child's face, starting from the nose downward,	Too loose a fit will not ensure adequate oxygen delivery.

Table 5.4. *(cont.)*

NURSING ACTIONS	RATIONALE
and adjust the nose clip and head strap (as described in Table 5.3, on the simple face mask).	
4. Document the method of oxygen delivery, the oxygen flow rate, and the child's response (respiratory effort, skin color, level of consciousness).	Communicates the nursing interventions and observations to health-care professionals.

TECHNIQUES TO SUPPORT VENTILATION

Generally, positive-pressure ventilation is used in emergency situations where the child's respiratory effort is insufficient. Positive-pressure ventilation can be administered by a bag-valve-mask device. When such equipment is not immediately available, mouth-to-mouth ventilation can be given using a pocket-type face mask.

Psychosocial Considerations

While the nonbreathing child requires immediate attention, the family's needs must also be considered. The parents' presence in the treatment room should be guided by hospital policy and by their ability to cope with the situation. If they are not in the treatment room, they should receive frequent updates of their child's condition by a member of the health-care team.

Mouth-to-Mouth Ventilation

Mouth-to-mouth ventilation is infrequently used in the hospital setting. Mouth-to-mouth ventilation is a reliable and effective method of ventilation, especially when the expired oxygen is supplemented with additional oxygen.

This method is difficult to administer in the presence of copious secretions, bleeding, or gastric regurgitation. Also, the increased awareness of transmittable infectious diseases has discouraged use of this technique by many health-care professionals.

Indications   Mouth-to-mouth ventilation is indicated in the infant or child with inadequate or no respiratory effort.

Contraindications   Possible meconium aspiration relative contraindications include vomiting, extensive facial trauma, bleeding.

Complications   Gastric distention; pneumothorax.

Equipment

> Gloves, goggles
> Pocket-type face mask

> Nursing responsibilities are described in Table 5.5.

Table 5.5. Nursing Responsibilities

NURSING ACTIONS	RATIONALE
1. Assess the child's respiratory effort and rate; don gloves and goggles.	
2. Open the airway, and assess for breathing. The airway can be opened by the head-tilt, chin-lift method (see Chapter 4), but only when there is no possibility of a cervical spine injury. If such an injury is suspected, use the jaw-thrust method. Both techniques displace the tongue anteriorly.	Opening the airway is of the utmost importance in children, as the tongue is frequently displaced into the posterior pharynx, occluding the airway. This measure alone may facilitate respiratory effort.[4]
3. If respiratory effort is absent or diminished, begin with the respiratory support procedures, and call for help. Use a pocket-type face mask or follow step 4.	If there is minimal or no response to assisted ventilations, the child will probably require placement of an artificial airway by an experienced person (see Chapter 4).
4. While awaiting help, cover the infant's mouth and nose with your mouth. In an older child, pinch the nose shut with your thumb and forefinger while maintaining head position; the child's mouth is then covered by your mouth.[4]	Obtains the best seal possible to enhance oxygen delivery.
5. After inhaling, give two small puffs of air for the infant; in the older child, more forceful exhalation may be required.	The breaths should be given slowly to ensure that adequate volume will be provided at the lowest pressure possible. This action will minimize the risk of gastric distention[4] and a pneumothorax.
6. If unable to ventilate, reposition the head and make another ventilation attempt.[4]	Improper airway positioning is the most common cause of airway obstruction,[4] thus repositioning is frequently helpful.
7. If the second attempt is still unsuccessful, initiate basic obstructed-airway maneuvers[4] (see Chapter 4).	
8. Following two ventilations, the child's pulse and respiratory status should be reevaluated and support continued if needed.	The child's normal, age-dependent respiratory rate must be taken into consideration.
9. If an oxygen source is available, the expired oxygen concentration can be increased about 16–17% by one of following: Place a nasal cannula on the resus-	Oxygen is, by far, the most important drug a child can receive. The drawback of mouth-to-mouth ventilation is reduced oxygen availability. A nasal cannula on the resuscitator

Table 5.5.   (*cont.*)

NURSING ACTIONS	RATIONALE
citator, and set the flow rate at 6 L/min.[5,6]	can increase the oxygen concentration to 30%.
	Oxygen tubing placed in the child's or the resuscitator's mouth can increase the oxygen concentration to 60%.
10. Place a nasogastric tube, as per physician order, if ventilation will be prolonged.	Many children will respond well to a brief period of assisted ventilation. If ventilation is prolonged, gastric distention is a potentially dangerous complication. Early placement of a nasogastric tube is desirable, to minimize this problem.
11. Reassess the airway and ventilatory status frequently, observe for complications, and document your actions.	Communicates the nursing interventions and observations to health-care professionals.

Bag-Valve-Mask Ventilation

The disadvantages of mouth-to-mouth ventilation are overcome by utilizing a bag-valve-mask type device. The bag-valve-mask device is used in conjunction with various airway adjuncts (e.g., oropharyngeal or nasopharyngeal airways) to facilitate ventilation.

Indications   Bag-valve-mask ventilation is indicated when inadequate or no respiratory effort is present.

Contraindications   Possible meconium aspiration.

Complications   Gastric distention, pneumothorax.

Equipment

> Ventilation bag-valve with oxygen reservoir
>> Neonatal bag (delivers a tidal volume up to 250 cc)
>> Pediatric bag (delivers a tidal volume up to 500 cc)
>> Adult bag (delivers a tidal volume of approximately 1500 cc)
> Masks: pediatric; neonate; infant; small adult; adult
> Gloves, goggles, mask
> Nonhumidified oxygen source
> Suction device
> Suction catheters (5 French — 14 French)
> Nasogastric tube

Nursing responsibilities are described in Table 5.6.

Table 5.6. Nursing Responsibilities

NURSING ACTIONS	RATIONALE
1. Assess the child's respiratory effort and rate; don gloves, goggles, mask.	
2. Obtain an appropriate size of ventilation bag-valve mask, and an oxygen delivery system. The ventilation bag-valve should be equipped with an oxygen reservoir; it should have a pop-off valve, which can be occluded. An appropriate bag-valve device delivers a tidal volume of 10–15 cc/kg during assisted ventilations.[1] Ensure that the mask fits the face securely. The mask should extend from the bridge of the nose to the cleft of the chin, enveloping the nose and mouth while avoiding compression of the eyes.[1] Ideally, masks should be clear, to allow for visualization of secretions and observation of the child's skin color.[1]	The reservoir bag allows for the administration of 60–90% oxygen, when the flow rate is set at 10–15 L/min with the neonatal or pediatric ventilation bag-valve; adult bags require flow rates of > 15 L/min.[1] Supplemental oxygen should always be administered to an unstable or potentially unstable child.[1,5] Many ventilation bags are equipped with a pressure-limited pop-off valve set at 35–45 cm H_2O, in an effort to reduce barotrauma.[1] Infants and children with poorly compliant lungs (due to drowning, hyaline membrane disease, etc.) or those receiving cardiopulmonary resuscitation (CPR) may require pressures that exceed the pop-off limit.[1] Mask leakage is a significant problem with this type of ventilation. In general, an inflatable mask provides a better seal, which improves ventilation.
3. Open the child's airway, and assess the child's breathing. The airway can be opened by the head-tilt, chin-lift method (see Chapter 4), but only when there is no possibility of a cervical spine injury. If such an injury is suspected, use the jaw-thrust method. Both of these methods displace the tongue anteriorly.	Opening the airway is imperative in children; frequently, the tongue is displaced into the posterior pharynx, occluding the airway. This measure alone may facilitate respiratory effort.
4. If respirations are inadequate or absent, firmly place a correctly sized mask over the child's mouth and nose with the thumb and second finger of one hand. The third finger is hooked around the angle and body of the mandible to displace the jaw upward (see Figure 5.3).	Proper mask positioning and head placement is critical to ensure delivery of an adequate tidal volume. Pulling the jaw forward will displace the tongue anteriorly.

Table 5.6. *(cont.)*

NURSING ACTIONS	RATIONALE

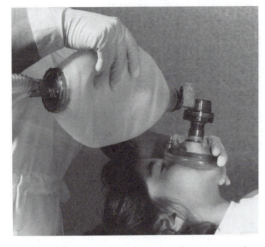

Figure 5.3. Correct hand placement for bag-valve-mask ventilation. Note that the mask makes a tight seal around the mouth and nose, with the jaw thrust forward slightly.

NURSING ACTIONS	RATIONALE
5. Deliver air slowly from the bag into the child's oropharynx; observe for chest expansion.	During bag compression, the gas intake valve closes, diverting oxygen to the reservoir. The fishmouth valve opens, forcing the flow of oxygen to the child.[1] During exhalation, the fishmouth valve closes, and the child's exhaled gases are vented into the atmosphere.[1]
6. Place a nasogastric tube, as per physician order, if ventilation will be prolonged.	Early placement of a nasogastric tube minimizes gastric distention. Gastric distention places pressure on the diaphragm, further compromising respiratory effort.
7. Document and assess the child's response to ventilation and the amount of time ventilation is assisted.	Many children will respond well to a brief period of assisted ventilation. Documentation communicates the nursing interventions and observations to health-care professionals.

CHEST DECOMPRESSION

Two potentially lethal complications of basic and advanced airway interventions are pneumothorax and hemothorax. Either of these conditions can interfere with the diffusion of oxygen and carbon dioxide at the alveolar level. Typically, these processes result from thoracic trauma; however, a variety of respiratory diseases of neonates and children can be complicated by a pneumothorax.

Children who present with a significant pneumothorax (greater than 10–20%) often have severe respiratory distress, evidenced by nasal flaring, tachypnea, sub/suprasternal retractions, tachycardia (progressing to bradycardia), and cyanosis. Breath sounds are usually decreased on the affected side.

Assisting with Needle Decompression of the Chest

While a simple pneumothorax may cause respiratory distress, progression to a *tension pneumothorax* (in which air accumulates in the pleural space and shifts the mediastinal structures thereby compressing the contralateral lung and decreasing cardiac output) is life-threatening.[7] There is seldom time for chest x-ray confirmation. Instead, the emergent placement of a large-bore catheter into the pleural space is indicated until tube thoracostomy is accomplished.

Indications   Needle decompression of the chest is indicated in a suspected tension pneumothorax: respiratory distress and hypotension, associated with increased jugular venous pressure, tracheal shift to the noneffected side (not always seen in children), decreased breath sounds and hyperresonance, subcutaneous emphysema increased central venous pressure (CVP), and pulsus paradoxus. Electromechanical disassociation and increased resistance to bag-valve ventilation (despite suctioning) may also indicate the presence of a significant pneumothorax.

Contraindications   Preceding criteria not met; trained personnel not available.

Complications   Lung injury, injury to the internal mammary artery (which is adjacent to the sternum), or intercostal vessel laceration. Such injuries can, in turn, lead to a significant hemothorax. Other complications include recurrent tension pneumothorax, which necessitates a second needle, and/or infection.

Equipment

> Needle
>> Older children: over-the-needle catheter (sizes 14–18 gauge)
>> Neonate/infant: butterfly needle (sizes 21–23 gauge) may be preferred
> 30- to 50-cc syringe and stopcock
> One-way flutter valve or extension tubing
> Small bottle of sterile water
> Povidone-iodine solution
> Gloves

Psychosocial Considerations   While needle decompression of the chest relieves respiratory distress, it may heighten the child's anxiety. The child (awake or unresponsive) should receive simple explanations of what will happen and what he or she will feel ("cold soap," "a pinch on your chest"). Consider turning the child's head away from the insertion site or shielding the child's eyes during the procedure, to decrease fear.

Explain to the parents what is happening and why. Take the time with them later to answer their questions and to clarify any misconceptions.

Nursing responsibilities are described in Table 5.7.

Table 5.7. Nursing Responsibilities

NURSING ACTIONS	RATIONALE
1. Assess the child's condition for signs of tension pneumothorax and notify an appropriate health professional.	A tension pneumothorax can be immediately relieved by needle decompression; ultimately, however, chest-tube placement is required.
2. Obtain the equipment listed herein; don gloves.	The over-the-needle catheter is the most common device for needle decompression and can be left in place for a short period of time. A butterfly needle, used in the neonate or infant, is removed after decompression. The stopcock is necessary to prevent a pleural leak and redevelopment of a tension pneumothorax while the syringe is being emptied of air. A flutter valve or extension tubing placed in a sterile bottle of water serves the same purpose, by creating an underwater seal and not allowing air to return to the pleural space.
3. Explain the procedure to the child and family, if time permits.	Enhances their understanding and cooperation. Time may not allow for this preparation.
4. The physician locates the second or third intercostal space (ICS), on the midclavicular line (MCL) on the affected side.[8]	The usual site for decompression of a tension pneumothorax is the second or third ICS, MCL due to the relative ease of access and the absence of significant structures.
5. The physician cleanses the skin with a povidone–iodine solution.	While needle decompression is generally done on an emergent basis, the skin should still be thoroughly prepared with antiseptic solution.
6. The physician inserts the catheter-over-needle device, with the syringe attached, into the second ICS, following the upper border of the third rib.	The intercostal artery and vein run along the inferior margin of each rib; thus, the needle should be inserted on the superior portion of the rib, to avoid injuring these vessels.[8]
7. Air will enter the syringe upon entry into the pleural space. The needle is then removed, and air is continually aspirated until no additional air can be aspirated into the syringe. Air will enter the syringe under pressure, which may cause the plunger to become separated from the syringe. If a syringe is not used, a gush of air will be felt from the catheter.	Relieves pneumothorax.
8. Following air removal, attach a one-way valve to the catheter hub, or	Some texts advise leaving the catheter open to atmospheric pressure,

Table 5.7. *(cont.)*

NURSING ACTIONS	RATIONALE
connect extension tubing to the hub, and place the end in a sterile water bottle, for an underwater seal.	thereby reducing a tension pneumothorax to an open pneumothorax. If the extension tubing method is used, bubbles will be noted in the water, verifying the presence of a tension pneumothorax.
9. Assist with tube thoracostomy as soon as possible. (See the following procedure.)	Needle decompression is a temporizing measure and should be followed by tube thoracostomy.
10. Document the time of the procedure and the child's response to the needle decompression; observe for a recurrence of pneumothorax.	Communicates the nursing interventions and observations to health-care professionals.

Assisting with Tube Thoracostomy

Chest tubes are used to treat a pneumothorax or hemothorax. Children who present initially with a tension pneumothorax can be managed for a short time with needle decompression; however, this procedure is not suited to long-term use.

Only about 15% of thoracic injuries require thoracostomy.[7] Nevertheless, every facility treating pediatric trauma patients should be prepared to diagnose and treat such injuries because these problems often occur in locations remote from a medical center or a thoracic surgeon.[7]

Indications   Tube thoracostomy is indicated in the presence of a tension pneumothorax, a moderate to large pneumothorax (> 10%), or any pneumothorax associated with significant respiratory symptoms.[9] Other indications for tube placement include bilateral pneumothoraces, associated hemothorax, need for mechanical ventilation in the presence of a pneumothorax, and increasing size of a pneumothorax despite initial therapy.[9]

Contraindications   Asymptomatic pneumothorax (< 10%); trained personnel not available.

Complications   Improper insertion of the tube, causing injury to the lung, liver, or diaphragm; injury to the neurovascular bundle, causing hemorrhage; air leak; and empyema.[9]

Equipment

> Chest tubes — sizes:[9]
>> Newborn   8–12 French
>> Infant   14–20 French
>> Child   20–28 French
>> Adolescent   28–42 French
> Local anesthetic

Various syringes and needles
Scalpel
Sterile curved clamps
Scissors
Underwater-seal collection system
Suture material
Tape
Petrolatum gauze
Gloves, goggles, mask

Psychosocial Considerations   This invasive procedure can create many fantasies in young children. They may believe that their insides are going to leak into the tube. The noise of the closed-chest draining system and the fluid collecting in the system may exacerbate this belief. Young children need repeated simple explanations and reassurance. Older children can be told what is happening in more detail because they have an understanding of how their bodies work. Ensure that the child receives a local anesthetic; sedation should be considered whenever possible. Consider turning the child's face away from the site or shielding the child's eyes during tube insertion to decrease fear. Help distract the child by concentrating on rhythmic breathing exercises.

Parents should probably not be present during chest-tube insertion, due to its invasiveness; however, each individual situation should be assessed. Nursing responsibilities are described in Table 5.8.

Table 5.8.   Nursing Responsibilities

NURSING ACTIONS	RATIONALE
1. Assess for a pneumothorax or hemothorax, and notify the appropriate health professional.	As noted, a careful respiratory assessment should be performed initially and reassessment done frequently.
2. Explain the procedure to the child and family, if time permits; seek additional assistance from personnel if needed.	Enhances their understanding and cooperation. Time may not allow for this preparation.
3. Obtain the equipment listed herein; don gloves.	When a hemothorax exists, the largest size of tube possible should be used, to ensure adequate drainage of blood.
4. Assist with injection of local anesthetic.	Puncture of the pleura is painful; thus, a local anesthesic should be available even for the unconscious child. This preparation may be eliminated in life-threatening situations or cardiac arrest.
5. The physician locates the site—the fourth or fifth ICS in the mid or anterior axillary line.[8,9]	In children, because they have wide diaphragmatic excursion, chest tubes are placed higher, to avoid inadvertent insertion of the tube into the abdominal cavity.[8]

Table 5.8. (*cont.*)

NURSING ACTIONS	RATIONALE
6. Help the physician prepare, drape, and infiltrate the area with a local anesthetic to the rib and along the subcutaneous tissue through which the tube will be tunneled.	
7. The physician incises the skin, usually 3–5 cm, with a scalpel, parallel to the long axis of the rib.[9]	
8. The physician bluntly dissects down to the rib with a clamp or scissors.[9] A clamp is curved over the superior edge of the rib, dividing the intercostal muscle down to the parietal pleura, which is penetrated.[9] The opening is enlarged by blunt dissection. A tunneling technique may be used to maintain the tube's position; this technique involves dissection across the intercostal space above the incision site and over the next rib.	Allows for visualization of the area for tube insertion.
9. The physician probes the opening with a finger in older infants and children.	Ensures that there are no adhesions of the lung and that the tube will be inserted into the chest and not subdiaphragmatically.[9]
10. Using a curved clamp, the physician grasps the chest tube at the tip and advances it through the tunnel and ICS into the chest, directing it posteriorly and apically.[9]	As with needle decompression, the interspace is entered superior to the rib, to avoid injury to the neurovascular bundle.
11. Connect the chest tube to an underwater seal; usually 15–25 cm water suction is used for a hemothorax or air leak.[9]	
12. The physician sutures the tube in place and dresses it with a sterile covering.	Often, the sterile covering is a petrolatum-type gauze, which is used as an air seal.[9]
13. Obtain a chest x-ray after the procedure, to confirm placement.	
14. Carefully measure the amount of blood from the chest tube.	A major hemothorax can rapidly result in hypovolemic shock and requires aggressive ventilatory and circulatory support, including crystalloids and blood products. Surgical intervention may be indicated if bleeding continues or worsens, or if it is impossible to evacuate adequately the retained blood from the pleural space.[7] Blood that is undrained within the pleural cavity can

Table 5.8. (*cont.*)

NURSING ACTIONS	RATIONALE
	lead to fibrothorax and, eventually, to scoliosis in the growing child.[7]
15. Document the time of the procedure, the size of chest tube, the amount of water suction, and the child's response to the procedure; observe for complications.	Communicates the nursing interventions and observations to health-care professionals.

Pulse Oximetry

Pulse oximetry uses light absorption to measure the percentage of arterial oxygenated hemoglobin.[10] Oxygen saturation is measured by comparing the amount of infrared light absorbed by deoxygenated hemoglobin with the amount of infrared light absorbed by oxygenated hemoglobin.[10] Each heartbeat produces swelling of tissue with oxygenated blood, and each pulse is sensed by the change in saturation between pulsations.

Pulse oximetry has several advantages.[10] First, it is noninvasive. Second, it does not use heated surfaces or require special site preparation. Third, under most conditions, it is accurate in the neonate, infant, child, and adult. Finally, results are immediately obtained.

Indications   Pulse oximetry is indicated when an infant or child requires continuous or intermittent measurement of arterial oxygenation and pulse rate. Examples include respiratory distress, sepsis, and hypovolemia; other indications include monitoring of sleep apnea, oxygen weaning, and pulmonary exercise testing. On occasion, it can be used as an alternative for painful, invasive arterial punctures.

Contraindications   In cases of severe hypoperfusion and vasoconstriction, the pulse oximeter may give inaccurate results. A more invasive technique, arterial puncture, should be used to assess oxygenation. Similarly, vasoactive drugs or intravascular dyes can pose a problem. A relative contraindication is development of an allergic reaction to the adhesive tape. Excessive movement, as often occurs with infants and children, can also cause inaccuracy of the measurements.

Complications   Impaired skin integrity, if used for greater than 8 hours.

Equipment

> Pulse oximeter
> Sensors
> Battery source

Psychosocial Considerations   Explain to the awake child that the sensor will feel like a Band-Aid™ on her or his finger. The child may relate the red glow to "ET—the Extraterrestrial." If appropriate, have the child sit on the parent's lap. This action may gain the child's cooperation and lessen anxiety.

Nursing responsibilities are described in Table 5.9.

Table 5.9. Nursing Responsibilities

NURSING ACTIONS	RATIONALE
1. Explain the procedure to the child and the family.	Enhances their understanding and cooperation.
2. Place the sensor on the index finger, as instructed by the manufacturer, and turn the machine on. Most sensors can also be applied to a thumb, smaller finger, or great toe. Sensors must be oriented as directed, or the values may be inaccurate. Avoid placing the sensor on any extremity with an arterial line, blood pressure cuff, or intravenous line in place. Restrain the extremity, as needed.	Wrapping the sensor too tightly around the digit may result in venous pulsations and an inaccurate reading.
3. Observe and record the pulse and the arterial saturation. If the sensor is not tracking the pulse reliably, check the position of the sensor.	Inability to obtain a readout may be due to incorrect positioning, or the sensor site may be too thick, thin, or deeply pigmented.
4. Document the child's response to the procedure and the pulse oximetry reading.	Communicates the nursing interventions and observations to health-care professionals.

REFERENCES

1. Chameides L, ed. Textbook of pediatric advanced life support. Dallas: American Academy of Pediatrics and American Heart Association, 1988:3–9, 11–19, 21–36.
2. Hughes TW, Buescher ES. Pediatric procedures. 2nd ed. Philadelphia: W.B. Saunders, 1980, 230.
3. Hunsinger DL, Lisnerski KJ, Maurizi JJ, Phillips ML. Respiratory technology procedure and equipment manual. Reston, VA: Reston Publishing Co., 1980;108, 111.
4. Albarran-Sotelo R, Flint LS, Kelly KJ, eds. Instructor's manual for basic life support. Dallas: American Heart Association, 1987: 65.
5. Secord-Pletz B. Resuscitation: Principles and techniques. In: Cosgriff JH, Anderson DL. The practice of emergency care. 2nd ed. Philadelphia: J.B. Lippincott, 1984;   .
6. Stewart R. Field airway control for the trauma patient. In: Campbell JF. Basic trauma life support. 2nd ed. Englewood Cliffs, NJ: Prentice-Hall, 1988;66.
7. Jones KW. Thoracic trauma. In: Mayer TA, ed. Emergency management of pediatric trauma. Philadelphia: W.B. Saunders, 1985:260, 254, 261.
8. Mayer TA. Initial evaluation and management of the injured child. In: Mayer TA, ed. Emergency management of pediatric trauma. Philadelphia: W.B. Saunders, 1985:20.
9. Barken RM, Rosen P. Emergency pediatrics. 3rd ed. St. Louis: C.V. Mosby, 1990;685–686.
10. Czervinske MP. Arterial blood gas analysis and other cardiopulmonary monitoring. In: Koff PB, Eitzman DV, Neu J. Neonatal and pediatric respiratory care. St. Louis: C.V. Mosby, 1988:260–281.

CHAPTER

6

Procedures Involving the Cardiovascular System

Sarah Martin

OVERVIEW OF PEDIATRIC CARDIOVASCULAR DIFFERENCES

There are several cardiovascular differences between the child and the adult. These differences include vital signs and cardiovascular functioning. Reference vital-sign values provide a comparison to the infant's or child's actual heart rate and blood pressure. However, the vital signs may not be the most appropriate indicators of the child's condition. Ongoing evaluation of the child is essential to detect subtle changes obtained by clinical assessment.

Age-appropriate heart-rate values are listed in Chapter 1, Table 1.1. Heart-rate values tend to decrease with age. As a general rule, a heart rate of 200 exceeds normal parameters. Systolic blood pressure can be estimated by age. For children over the age of 2 years, the approximate 50th percentile for systolic blood pressure equals 90 + (2 × age in years),[1] while the lower limit for systolic blood pressure is approximated by 70 + (2 × age in years).[1]

A child with decreased cardiovascular function exhibits signs of decreased cardiac output. As in adults, cardiac output equals the heart rate times the stroke volume. Cardiac output reflects the volume of blood pumped by the heart per minute.[1]

Stroke volume can be improved by increasing cardiac preload, increasing ventricular contractility, and reducing ventricular afterload.[2] Stroke volume increases with age.[2]

Optimal preload is achieved by appropriate intravenous (IV) fluid administration.[2] Maintenance of electrolyte balance and acid–base status improves myocardial contractility.[2] In children, calcium, potassium, glucose, and arterial blood gas determinations should be performed frequently. Afterload can be optimized pharmacologically with β_2-adrenergic agents and drugs with vasodilatory effects.

Preload, myocardial contractility, and afterload are evaluated with invasive hemodynamic monitoring and clinical observation. The child with decreased cardiac output demonstrates inadequate end-organ perfusion. Decreased cardiac output is demonstrated by cool peripheral temperature, warm core temperature, mottled extremities, tachycardia, weak pulse, sluggish capillary refill, decreased level of consciousness, and decreased urine output (< 1 cc/kg/hour).[1,2,3,4] Late signs of cardiac failure include hypotension, metabolic acidosis, and bradycardia.[2,4,5] Hypovolemic shock is the most common form of shock in the pediatric trauma patient.[4] Often, the obvious signs of hypovolemic shock develop late. In children, there may be a 15–20% loss of circulating blood volume before signs of shock develop.[5] Children have an exaggerated release of catecholamines (endogenous epinephrine and norepinephrine) with blood loss, with a resultant vasoconstriction and maintenance of systolic blood pressure.[4]

Children have a higher circulating blood volume per unit of body weight, as compared to adults.[3] A child's circulating blood volume is approximately 75 mL/kg.[3] For hypotension to occur, the child must lose 30–40% of his or her circulating blood volume.[4]

Careful and continuous assessment of cardiovascular parameters is necessary to intervene appropriately with an infant or child presenting to the emergency department for treatment.

NONINVASIVE MONITORING

Cardiac Monitoring

Indications   Noninvasive cardiac monitoring allows for continuous monitoring of the electrocardiogram (ECG) and respiratory rate. It is indicated for evaluating cardiac dysrhythmias, heart rate, respiratory rate, and respiratory pattern. Noninvasive cardiac monitoring is also useful as an adjunct to clinical assessment of infants and children at risk for cardiac or respiratory instability.

Contraindications   None.

Complications   Skin irritation from electrode gel.

Equipment

>   Neonate-size electrodes
>   Child-size electrodes
>   Adult-size electrodes
>   Alcohol wipes
>   Standard three-lead cable
>   Cardiac/respiratory monitor

Psychosocial Considerations   Young children may fantasize about the cardiac monitor's function. Explain that the electrodes do not hurt and that these "stickers on the chest" allow the machine to measure their heartbeats. Older children may appreciate having a rhythm strip as they have a basic understanding of how the heart works.

Parents need to know the indications for cardiac monitoring. The family may become focused on the monitor's rhythm display, beeping, and alarming. They may need help to focus on their child's needs and not on the cardiac monitor.

Nursing responsibilities are described in Table 6.1.

Table 6.1. Nursing Responsibilities

NURSING ACTIONS	RATIONALE
1. Explain to the child and the family why the cardiac monitor is needed.	Enhances their understanding and cooperation.
2. Swab the child's skin with alcohol wipes where the electrodes will be placed. Let the skin dry.	Ensures cleanliness of skin for good skin–electrode contact.
3. Place the appropriate size of electrodes for monitoring of standard ECG. The neonatal size is used in newborns and young infants. The pediatric size is used in older infants through early school age children. Adult size electrodes are used in older children and adolescents.	Allows for proper electrical conduction. Maximizes available skin surface.
4. When applying the electrodes, press firmly from the outer edge toward the center. For a three-lead ECG:	Keeps conductive gel in the center; prevents skin breakdown or discomfort when removing the electrodes.
a. The negative electrode ("RA" or "right arm") is placed at the second intercostal space, right midclavicular line. Avoid the nipple area with the electrode placement.[6]	

b. The positive electrode ("LA" or "left arm") is placed at the fourth intercostal space, in the left anterior axillary line.[6]	Negative or positive is determined by lead selection on the cardiac monitor such that
	
	Lead I: RA is negative
	          LA is positive
	Lead II: RA is negative
	           LL is positive
	Lead III: LA is negative
	            LL is positive
	Usually, lead II provides the most upright P, R, and T waveforms.

c. The ground electrode ("LL" or "leg") is placed in the sixth intercostal space, anterior axillary line.	The third electrode acts as a ground in a three-lead system.
5. Set high/low alarms.	Detects changes in cardiac rate.
6. Observe and assess ECG tracing.	Allows for appropriate cardiac rhythm evaluation.
7. Offer a sample tracing to the child.	
8. Record the ECG tracing and place it on the child's Emergency Depart-	Communicates the nursing interventions and observations to health-care

Table 6.1.   *(cont.)*

NURSING ACTIONS	RATIONALE
ment record. Analyze the ECG tracing for rate and rhythm (see Figure 6.1).	professionals.

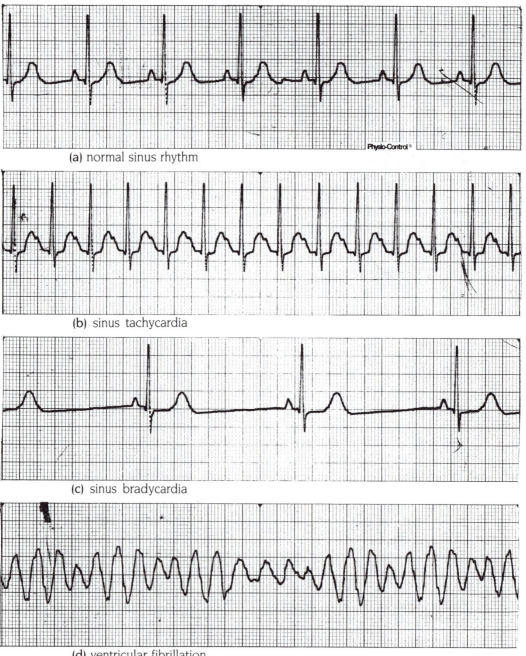

(a) normal sinus rhythm

(b) sinus tachycardia

(c) sinus bradycardia

(d) ventricular fibrillation

Figure 6.1. Common electrocardiogram readings in children (a) normal sinus rhythm; (b) sinus tachycardia; (c) sinus bradycardia; (d) ventricular fibrillation.

Twelve-Lead Electrocardiogram (ECG)

Indications   A 12-lead ECG is indicated in children with cardiac dysrhythmias, ingestions/poisonings, syncopal episodes, chest trauma, and known or suspected congenital heart disease.

Contraindications   None known.

Complications   Skin irritation from conductive cream.

Equipment

> ECG machine with paper
> Patient cable with one chest and four limb wires
> Four limb cables with alligator clips (if indicated for use with machine); one chest cable with suction cup or alligator clips
> Four limb electrodes and eight chest electrodes (neonatal or pediatric); for use with alligator clips or conductive cream

Psychosocial Considerations   When explaining this procedure to the young child, tell the child that "you will make a drawing without using crayons or pencils with these stickers (electrodes) or bracelets (limb cables)." Allow the child to examine the conductive cream or the suction cup for chest leads (if used), to help allay anxiety and gain trust. Support the child by giving him or her a small segment of a rhythm strip. School-age and adolescent females may be embarrassed when exposing their chest for the procedure. Assure their privacy.

Nursing responsibilities are described in Table 6.2.

Table 6.2.   Nursing Responsibilities

NURSING ACTIONS	RATIONALE
1. Explain to the child and the family the need for the ECG.	Enhances their understanding and cooperation.
2. Provide comfort measures for the child, such as keeping the room warm, minimizing chest exposure, and maintaining privacy.	Minimizes artifact because loose electrode connections, broken lead wire, and the child's movement can cause artifact.
3. Place an electrode or conductive cream distally on each extremity. Limb electrodes should be placed on fleshy areas.	
4. Place six chest electrodes with conductive cream.[7]	Inappropriate wire placement provides erroneous information.
V_1: Fourth intercostal space at right sternal border	
V_2: Fourth intercostal space at left sternal border	
V_3: Midway between V_2 and V_4— left chest (often omitted)	
V_4: Left fifth intercostal space at midclavicular line	

Table 6.2.   *(cont.)*

NURSING ACTIONS	RATIONALE
V$_5$: Left anterior axillary line lateral to V$_4$	
V$_6$: Left midaxillary line lateral to V$_5$	
V$_4$R: Right fifth intercostal space at the midclavicular line (often omitted)	
V$_3$R: Midway between V$_4$R and V$_1$—right chest	V$_3$R is added to provide an extra view of the electrical forces from the right side of the heart.[6]
5. Attach cable wires to appropriate extremity. Cable wires are labeled RA = right arm, LA = left arm, RL = right leg, and LL = left leg.	
6. Prepare the machine for recording. Place the recording stylus in the center of the paper. Set the chart speed at 25 mm/second. Place in automatic mode, if available.	Standard ECG paper speed; 1 mm (a small square) represents 0.04 seconds, and 5 mm (a large square) represents 0.2 seconds.
7. Initiate ECG recording, with limb leads progressing to chest leads. Most machines will automatically record 2.8-second strips of lead I through avF. A lead II rhythm strip of longer duration may be needed for rhythm analysis. Adjust placement of the chest wire by moving the alligator clip or suction cup.	
8. The ECG machine marks the ECG paper according to a standard marking code.	
9. Give the child a sample ECG tracing to take home.	
10. Document the child's name, date, and time on the ECG tracing. Interpret the tracing.	Communicates the nursing interventions and observations to health-care professionals.

Blood Pressure Measurement

Indications   Blood pressure (BP) measurement is indicated to provide noninvasive assessment of the infant's and child's systemic perfusion.

Contraindications   BP measurements are not obtained in extremities with uncompromised neurovascular integrity.

Complications   None known; hematoma if the child has bleeding tendencies.

Equipment

> Appropriate size of BP cuff and sphygmomanometer
> Stethoscope
> Doppler
> Aqueous coupling gel (for Doppler use)
> Automated BP monitor

Psychosocial Considerations   Young children may believe that their BP is something that is "taken" from them. Children usually do not like the pressure around their arm or the tingling in their fingers during this procedure. Use phrases that are noninvasive, such as "measure your blood pressure" or "give your arm a hug." Give the child something to do while the BP is being measured (look at mercury column, wiggle fingers, count, hold something in her or his other hand, pump up the cuff). Praise the child for holding his or her arm still. Parents can assist by holding children on their lap to help them feel secure. It might also help to demonstrate the technique on a doll or the parent beforehand to prepare the child for the procedure.

Nursing Responsibilities

Standard Measurement   Nursing responsibilities are described in Table 6.3.

Table 6.3.   Nursing Responsibilities

NURSING ACTIONS	RATIONALE
1. Explain to the child and the family why the BP needs to be measured. Tell the child what he or she will feel; "This cuff will give your arm a hug."	Enhances their understanding and cooperation.
2. Place the infant or child in a comfortable position, such as sitting on the parent's lap.	May calm the child and allow for more accurate BP measurement.
3. Select the appropriate size of BP cuff. Cuff size applies to the inner bladder, not the cloth covering. The cuff should cover 75% of the upper arm, and the bladder should be over the artery, encircling half of the limb (see Figure 6.2). Data are lacking for determination of the appropriate size of cuff for lower-extremity use.[9]	Cuffs that are too wide provide falsely low readings. Cuff that are too narrow yield falsely high readings.

Table 6.3.   *(cont.)*

NURSING ACTIONS	RATIONALE

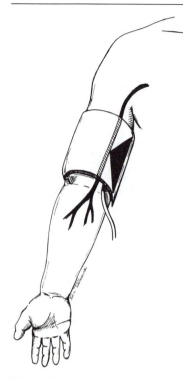

Figure 6.2. Proper size and position of blood pressure (BP) cuff. To obtain proper compression of the brachial artery, the cuff should encircle two thirds of the upper arm, approximately 1 inch from the antecubital fossa, with the bladder centered over the brachial artery.

4. Apply the cuff snugly to the extremity (upper arm or thigh). The lower edge of the cuff should be 1 inch above the palpated pulse.

   Allows for accurate measurement.

5. Palpate the artery distal to the cuff (brachial or popliteal artery).

   Determines correct placement for auscultation.

6. Place the diaphragm or bell of the stethoscope over the area where the pulse was palpated. During the first assessment, palpate the pulse on inflation, and auscultate on deflation. Subsequent measurements may be done using previous systolic pressure to determine top inflation pressure.

   Allows for adequate sound transmission.

7. Inflate the cuff 20 mm Hg above the pressure at which the arterial pulsation disappears.[8]

   Provides enough pressure to compress the artery.

Table 6.3.   (*cont.*)

NURSING ACTIONS	RATIONALE
8. Auscultate while deflating the cuff at a rate of 2–3 mm Hg per second.[8] If a repeat BP is needed, wait 30 seconds after the cuff is fully deflated.	Ensures accuracy of measurement, as too rapid or too slow deflation may yield inaccurate readings.[8]
9. Document the BP obtained.	Communicates nursing interventions and observations to health-care professionals.

Doppler   Nursing responsibilities are described in Table 6.4.

Table 6.4.   Nursing Responsibilities

NURSING ACTIONS	RATIONALE
1. Place the flat side of the transducer (filled with aqueous gel) over the artery distal to the cuff.	Permits measurement of BP in infants or children with poor perfusion or hypotension.
2. Inflate the BP cuff until the Doppler tones are not audible.	Pressure level occludes the artery, and ultrasound waves are reflected with no change in frequency.[9]
3. Deflate the cuff at a rate of 2–3 mm Hg per second.	Vessel opens with a change in frequency of reflected waves.[9]
4. Document the BP obtained (e.g., 90/D). Systolic BP is read as the initial tapping sounds are heard.	Alteration in frequency and pitch of the audible sound varies with the velocity of blood flow.

Palpation   Nursing responsibilities are described in Table 6.5.

Table 6.5.   Nursing Responsibilities

NURSING ACTIONS	RATIONALE
1. Palpate the brachial artery or popliteal artery.[9]	
2. Inflate the BP cuff to the point at which the arterial pulse is not palpable.[9]	
3. Deflate the cuff at a rate of 2–3 mm Hg per second.	
4. Document the BP obtained (e.g., 90/P). Systolic BP is recorded as the pressure at which the pulse is palpated.	Communicates the nursing interventions and observations to health-care professionals.

INTRAVENOUS CANNULATION/PHLEBOTOMY

Indications   Intravenous cannulation is indicated for fluid administration, medication administration, and access for obtaining venous blood samples.

Contraindications   Not performed in poorly perfused, infected, or burned sites.

Complications   Fluid overload, infiltration, phlebitis, air embolus, hematoma, thrombus.[1,10]

Equipment

> Phlebotomy:[1]
>> Butterfly needle
>>> 21, 23, 25 gauge: infants < 1 year
>>> 16, 18, 20 gauge: children 1–12 years
>>> 16, 18, 20 gauge: children > 12 years
>> Cannulation:[1]
>>> Over-the-needle catheter
>>>> 20, 22, 24 gauge: infants < 1 year
>>>> 16, 18, 20 gauge: children 1–12 years
>>>> 14, 16, 18 gauge: children > 12 years
> Tourniquet or rubber band (for scalp veins)
> Povidone–iodine solution
> Alcohol wipes
> One 3-cc syringe (for flush)
> Normal saline (NS)
> T-connector
> Tape
> Padded armboards (infant, pediatric, or adult size)
> Protective covering
> Razor for scalp vein insertion
> Gloves
> 2 × 2 sterile gauze, and tape, or transparent dressing
> IV infusion set-up (assembled)
> IV infusion pump recommended
> Tranoilluminator (optional)

Psychosocial Considerations   In the emergency department IV cannulation is undertaken frequently. Avoid cannulating the infant's and toddler's dominant (sucking) hand because sucking provides self comfort. When the hand or arm is secured with tape and an IV board, the young child will need time to assimilate this change. The child may try to remove the IV board; he or she should be given something else to hold or play with, if well enough to do so. The child may have a sense of control if allowed to decorate the protective cover with Band-Aid™s or stickers.

The child needs simple explanations and reassurances of what will happen ("I'm going to put this tube in your hand") and how it will feel ("a pinch"). Avoid saying "IV" as the young child may misinterpret "IV" as "ivy." The older child can be given the explanations of where the IV fluid goes and why it is needed.

Parents should have the option of staying or leaving during this procedure. They should not be asked to restrain the child, but they should be asked to comfort the child if they do stay.

Nursing responsibilities are described in Table 6.6.

Table 6.6. Nursing Responsibilities

NURSING ACTIONS	RATIONALE
1. Explain to the child and the family the need for venous cannulation, if time permits.	Enhances their understanding and cooperation.
2. Assemble the necessary equipment at the child's bedside.	Selection of an IV device depends on the vein location and the type of fluid or medication to be administered.[1]
3. Prepare tape for immobilizing the extremity and securing the catheter.	
4. Wash your hands.	Prevents spread of infection.
5. Select the appropriate size of cannulation device by evaluating venous access and available IV catheters.	Allows for ease of insertion.
6. Select an appropriate site. Utilize distal sites first. Avoid inserting the catheter near joints, at sites that limit mobility, and the dominant hand. Scalp and foot veins may be used in infants.	In infants, scalp and foot veins may be easy to visualize, due to limited subcutaneous fat.
7. Stabilize the selected site on a padded arm board or have another nurse immobilize the site (see Figure 6.3a).	Assists with proper immobilization to facilitate ease of insertion.

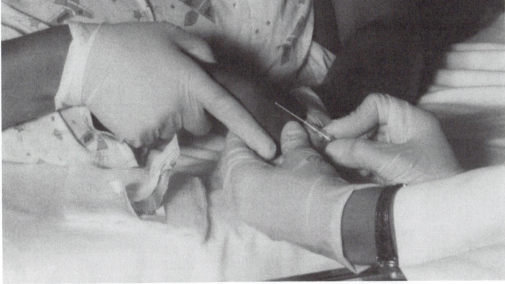

Figure 6.3.   (a) Positioning the hand for cannulation.

Table 6.6. (cont.)

NURSING ACTIONS	RATIONALE
8. Don clean gloves.	Complies with universal precautions.
9. Apply the tourniquet proximal to the insertion site. Place an open piece of gauze under the tourniquet. Rubber bands can be used as a tourniquet for scalp veins.[1]	Ensures that the tourniquet impedes venous flow, not arterial flow.[10] Gauze application prevents pinching the skin or pulling the hairs.
10. After the site is selected, remove the tourniquet.	Extreme or prolonged pressure may make the vein torturous.[10]
11. Reapply the tourniquet proximal to the site.	
12. Cleanse the site with a povidone–iodine solution.	Good infection control practice.
13. Wipe off povidone–iodine with an alcohol wipe; wait briefly after alcohol application.	Allows for visualization of vein. May prevent stinging on insertion.
14. Follow the procedures for either the butterfly needle or the over-the-needle catheter. (See Tables 6.7 and 6.8, respectively.) If unsuccessful after two attempts, summon assistance from another qualified health-care professional; use a new butterfly or over-the-needle catheter with each attempt.	Avoids prolonged discomfort. Allows child recovery time and ensures timely placement of IV device.
15. Calculate IV fluids for administration. Send blood specimens for analysis.	Ensures proper fluid management; ensures timely laboratory analysis.
16. Praise the child.	
17. Document the site of the catheter insertion, the size of the catheter, the type and rate of IV fluid administration, blood specimens obtained and how the child tolerated the procedure.	Communicates the nursing interventions and observations to health-care professionals.

Table 6.7. Nursing Responsibilities for Butterfly-Needle Phlebotomy

NURSING ACTIONS	RATIONALE
1. Do not flush the butterfly if it is to be used for drawing blood specimens. Flush after obtaining blood return, as small veins may clot off the butterfly-needle.	Avoids diluting and possibly contaminating the blood specimen.
2. Grasp the wings with the thumb and index finger.	Assists with manipulating the needle.

Table 6.7.   *(cont.)*

NURSING ACTIONS	RATIONALE
3. With the bevel upward, pull the skin distal to the site taut, and insert the needle into the vein, keeping the needle nearly parallel to the skin.	Assists in cannulating the vein.
4. Confirm placement by observing a blood return in the butterfly tubing.	
5. Remove the tourniquet.	
6. For phlebotomy, draw off the blood sample, remove the butterfly needle, and apply pressure with a 2 × 2 gauze pad.	
7. If the butterfly is to be used in fluid administration, securely tape it in place. Place a protective cover over the site.	Prevents accidental dislodgement of the butterfly.
8. Calculate IV fluids for administration. Send blood specimens for analysis.	Ensures proper fluid management; ensures timely laboratory analysis.
9. Praise the child.	
10. Document the site of the catheter insertion, the size of the catheter, the type and rate of IV fluid administration, blood specimens obtained and how the child tolerated the procedure.	Communicates the nursing interventions and observations to health-care professionals.

Table 6.8.   Nursing Responsibilities for Over-the-Needle Catheter

NURSING ACTIONS	RATIONALE
1. If desired, flush a T-connector and IV catheter with saline. Do not flush if blood specimens will be obtained.	
2. Pull the skin tight, distal to the insertion site.	Assists in cannulating the vein.
3. Insert the needle with the bevel up, at a 45° angle[10] (see Figure 6.3,b.).	Allows for smooth cannulation.

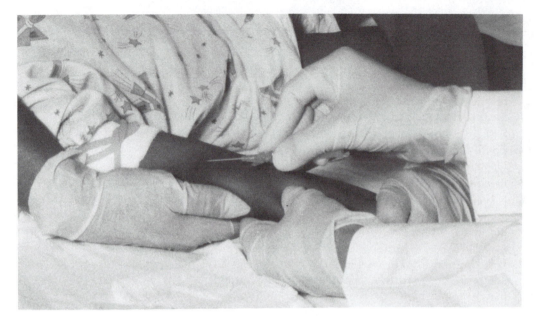

Figure 6.3.   (b) positioning the antecubital fossa for cannulation.

Table 6.8.   (*cont.*)

NURSING ACTIONS	RATIONALE
4. Reducing the angle, slowly advance the needle a few millimeters.[10]	
5. When a blood return is observed, advance the cannula while withdrawing the needle. Do not reinsert the needle into the catheter after it is removed.	Avoids puncture or shear of the cannula, caused by reintroduction of the needle.
6. Remove the tourniquet.	
7. Attach the T-connector, and obtain the blood specimen, if needed.	The T-connector facilitates taping of the tubing, securing of the needle, and changing of IV fluids without dislodging the catheter.
8. Flush the catheter.	Confirms catheter placement.
9. Tape the catheter securely in place. Place protective cover as needed (see Figures 6.4, 6.5, 6.6).	Prevents accidental dislodgement of the catheter.
10. Calculate IV fluids for administration. Send blood specimens for analysis.	Ensures proper fluid management; ensures timely laboratory analysis.
11. Praise the child.	
12. Document the site of the catheter insertion, the size of the catheter, the type and rate of IV fluid administration, blood specimens obtained and how the child tolerated the procedure.	Communicates the nursing interventions and observations to health-care professionals.

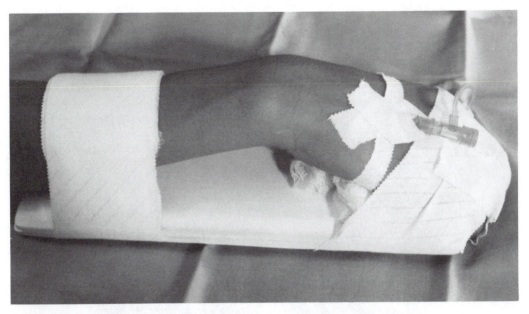

Figure 6.4.   An IV site is secure.

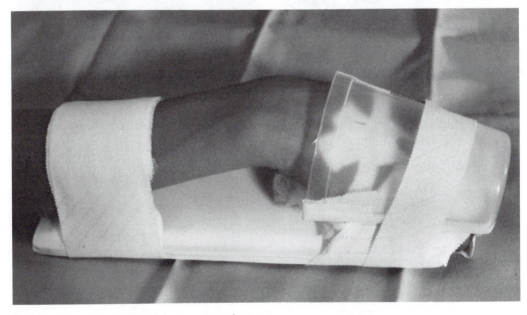

Figure 6.5.   A protective device is in place.

INTRAOSSEOUS INFUSION

The intraosseous (IO) technique provides an alternative method of venous access via the bone marrow. IO provides access to the systemic circulation when there is peripheral circulatory collapse.[11]

Indications   The IO route is indicated for the administration of fluids and/or medications in emergent situations[1] in children 6 years of age or younger.

Contraindications   Bone disorders, such as osteogenesis imperfecta and osteoporosis. The IO route should not be used in an extremity with local cellulitis, infected burns, or a fracture.[11]

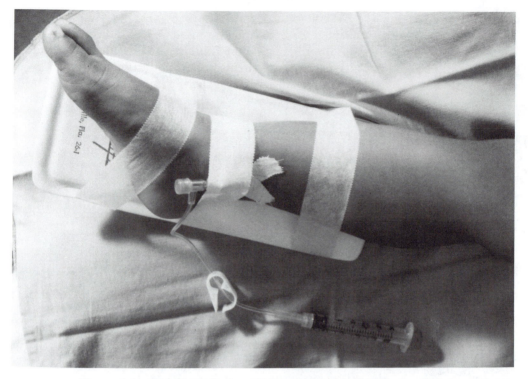

Figure 6.6. Stabilization of an IV (intravenous) catheter placed in the saphenous vein; extra taping over the foot arch may be necessary.

Complications   Osteomyelitis, subcutaneous abscess, extravasation of fluid into subcutaneous tissue, piercing of bone cortices, damage to the epiphysis, and fat embolism.[11,12]

Equipment

> Appropriate size of needle with stylet
>> Rosenthal bone-marrow needle or spinal needle
>>> 18-gauge: < 3 months of age
>>> 15-gauge: 3 months to 5 years
>>> 13-gauge: > 5 years
>> Jamshidi® sternal/iliac aspiration needle
>>> 18-gauge: < 3 months
>>> 15-gauge: > 3 months
>> Cook™ intraosseous access needle
> Povidone–iodine solution
> Three 5-cc syringes
> 1% lidocaine for local anesthetic (if needed)
> Normal saline flush
> Tape
> Padded arm board
> Gloves
> Fluid or medication to be infused
> Pressure infuser
> 2 × 2 gauze

Psychosocial Considerations   Explain to the awake or unconscious child what he or she will feel during the procedure. The family needs simple, direct explanations of their child's condition and proposed interventions. Parental presence should be guided by hospital policy, parents' coping abilities and the staff's preference. If the family chooses to remain in the treatment room, a designated staff support person should remain with them to tend to their needs.

Nursing responsibilities are described in Table 6.9.

Table 6.9.   Nursing Responsibilities

NURSING ACTIONS	RATIONALE
1. Explain to the child and the family the need for the IO infusion. Time may not allow for this preparation.	Enhances their understanding and cooperation.
2. Assist in administering a local anesthetic to the awake child.[11]	Minimizes discomfort during the procedure.
3. Support and immobilize the extremity.	Facilitates insertion of needle.
4. Apply povidone–iodine solution to the insertion site.[11,14]	Prevents infection.
5. Select an appropriate site.	Avoids risk of inserting the needle into the epiphyseal plate. Landmarks are easily identifiable with absence of intervening blood vessels and nerves.[11]
a. The preferred site is the flat anteriomedial surface of the proximal tibia in children, approximately 1–3 cm below the tibial tuberosity.[1,11,12] However, this site becomes harder to penetrate in the child over 6 years of age[11] (see Figure 6.7).	
b. Any marrow-containing cavity may be used (distal femur, distal tibia, iliac crest, sternum).[14,15]	Use of the sternum is discouraged because this site is too thin to guarantee safe placement.[15]
6. Insert the needle at a 30–45° angle with the bevel directed away from the epiphyseal plate,[15] using a rotary motion. When the needle passes through the cortex, the resistance decreases.	The tip of the needle should lie in the medullary cavity where marrow sinusoids drain into large medullary venous channels.[15]
7. Confirm the needle placement.	Proper placement decreases the chance of extravasation of fluids or medications.
a. A marrow aspirate may or may not be obtained.	
b. Flush with 2–3 cc of normal saline; minimal resistance should be met.	
c. The needle should stand unsupported.	
8. Infuse fluids or medications via a	

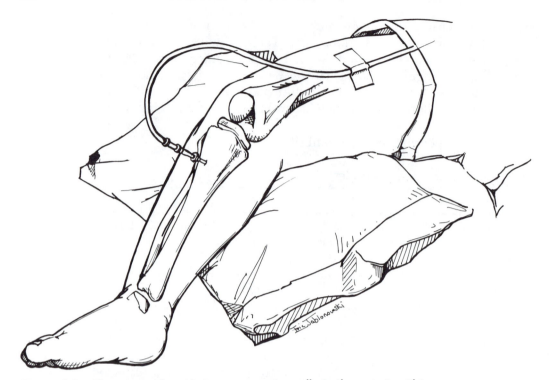

Figure 6.7.   Placement of an IO (intraosseous) needle in the anterior tibia.

Table 6.9.   *(cont.)*

NURSING ACTIONS	RATIONALE
standard IV setup or manually with a syringe. Use a pressure infusor[14] for rapid infusion.	
9. Document the site, needle size, and the child's response to the procedure.	Communicates the nursing interventions and observations to health-care professionals.
10. Discontinue the IO device when conventional IV access is obtained. IO access is intended for short-term use (less than 8 hours).	Minimizes associated complications.
11. Apply a sterile dressing after the IO device is discontinued.	Prevents infection.

ASSISTING WITH ARTERIAL CANNULATION

Indications   Arterial cannulation is indicated in children who are hypotensive or hypertensive, who are receiving vasoactive drugs, and who require frequent arterial blood sampling.

Contraindications   Arterial cannulation should not be performed in extremities where perfusion is compromised.

Complications   Air or particulate embolization, infection, inadvertent injection of a sclerosing agent,[1] exsanguination from inadvertent disconnection of the closed system.

Equipment

IV catheter
   Infants and children < 8 years — 22–24-gauge
   Children > 8 years — 20- 22-gauge
Povidone–iodine solution
Alcohol wipes
One 3-cc syringe with 25-gauge needle for local anesthetic
Local anesthetic (1% or 2% lidocaine, per physician preference)
Three 3-cc syringes (one for flush, one for discard sample, one for blood sample)
One 3-cc heparinized syringe for blood gas sample
Tape
Soft restraints
4 × 4 gauze
Heparinized saline (0.2 NS, 0.45 NS, 0.9 NS) solution
Padded arm board
1 pair of sterile gloves
1 pair of clean gloves
Dressing materials: 2 × 2 sterile gauze and tape, or transparent dressing
Transducer
Arterial pressure monitoring kit (assembled)
IV infusion pump or intraflow with pressure bag
Suture material (optional)
Goggles

Psychosocial Considerations   Explain to the awake or unconscious child what he or she will feel during the procedure. The family needs simple, direct explanations of their child's condition and proposed interventions. Parental presence should be guided by hospital policy, parents' coping abilities and staff's preference. If the family chooses to remain in the treatment room, a designated staff support person should remain with them to tend to their needs.

Nursing responsibilities are described in Table 6.10.

Table 6.10.   Nursing Responsibilities

NURSING ACTIONS	RATIONALE
1. Explain to the child and the family the need for arterial cannulation. Time may not allow for this preparation.	Enhances their understanding and cooperation.
2. Assemble the equipment at the child's bedside.	Allows for timely completion of the procedure.
3. Assemble and flush the arterial pressure monitoring system prior to cannulation.	
4. Assist the physician with selecting an appropriate arterial site for cannula-	If the radial, dorsalis pedis, posterior tibial, and femoral arteries cannot

Table 6.10. *(cont.)*

NURSING ACTIONS	RATIONALE
tion. Commonly used arteries include the radial, femoral, dorsalis pedis, and posterior tibial.[1] The axillary artery also can be used.[16]	be cannulated, the axillary artery should be considered.
5. Assess the extremity for adequate perfusion.	
a. If the *radial artery* is selected, the Allen test or a modified Allen test is performed. To perform the Allen test, maintain pressure on the radial and ulnar arteries at the wrist. If possible, have the child squeeze her or his fist until the hand blanches. Release the pressure on the ulnar artery,[17] and observe for flushing.	Flushing indicates that blood flow from the ulnar artery alone is adequate to perfuse the hand.
b. If the *dorsalis pedis* site is selected, place pressure on the pedal artery at the ankle or at the dorsalis pedis site. Compress the toenail of the great toe. Release the pressure, and observe for a return of color.	The return of color indicates adequate collateral flow.
6. Secure the arm or foot on an armboard. All digits should be visible.	Allows for assessment of peripheral perfusion.
7. Restrain the arms and legs as necessary.	Promotes safety and assists with cannulation.
8. Don clean gloves and goggles.	Complies with universal precautions.
9. Cleanse the skin with povidone–iodine solution.	Prevents infection.
10. Assist the physician in anesthetizing the skin with a local anesthetic.	Decreases pain during the procedure; may prevent arteriospasm.
11. Assist the physician with cannulation. Use sterile technique. After cannulation, connect the catheter to the arterial pressure monitoring system, and attach to a monitor.	Cannulation of arteries is a physician's responsibility. Assess for decannulation and inadvertent loose connections.
12. For the flush system, heparinized saline should be infused at 1 cc to 3 cc per hour.	Heparinized saline solution maintains patency of the high-pressure arterial system.[18]
13. Observe for an arterial waveform on the monitor. Normal characteristics of a waveform include initial sharp rise, slightly rounded top, and a dicrotic notch on the downslope and a tapering off of the downslope after	Assures adequate functioning of the arterial line. The dicrotic notch indicates start of diastole and closure of the aortic valve. The closer the arterial line is to the heart, the closer is the dicrotic notch to the top of the

Table 6.10.   *(cont.)*

NURSING ACTIONS	RATIONALE
the dicrotic notch.[17] Apply a sterile dressing.	curve.
14. Discontinue the catheter if there are signs of decreased perfusion, such as delayed capillary refill, coolness of the extremity, or mottling,[17] or if the child complains of tingling.	Blanching and a cool extremity distal to the catheter site indicate tissue damage.
15. After removing the catheter, apply direct pressure for 5–10 minutes, then apply a pressure dressing for 20–30 minutes.[17] The pressure dressing should never be circumferential.	Pressure aids in preventing hematoma formation,[17] but circumferential pressure impedes circulation.
16. Document the results of the Allen test, as well as the insertion site, the catheter size, the type of infusion, and the rate of infusion. Document the arterial and cuff blood pressures. Document how the child tolerated the procedure.	Communicates the nursing interventions and observations to health-care professionals.

ASSISTING WITH VENOUS CUTDOWN

Indications   Venous cutdown is indicated for fluid and medication administration when percutaneous, central, peripheral or IO access is unobtainable. Venous cutdown is a more stable means of venous access even if an IO device is in place.

Contraindications   Not performed in poorly perfused, infected, or burned extremities.

Complications   Cellulitis, thrombosis, hematoma, phlebitis, and catheter fragment embolism.

Equipment

> Over-the-needle catheters[1]
>> 20, 22, 24 gauge: infants < 1 year
>> 16, 18, 20 gauge: children 1–12 years
>> 14, 16, 18 gauge: children > 12 years
> Tourniquet
> Povidone–iodine solution
> 3-cc syringe with 25-gauge needle for local anesthetic
> Local anesthetic (1% or 2% lidocaine without epinephrine)
> 3-cc syringe (for flush)
> Normal saline
> T-connector
> Tape
> Padded arm board
> Soft restraints
> Protective covering

Cutdown tray
Suture material
Scalpel blade
Sterile draping towels
Sterile gloves, goggles
Dressing materials: 2 × 2 sterile gauze and tape, or transparent dressing
IV infusion setup (assembled)
IV infusion pump (recommended)

Psychosocial Considerations   Explain to the awake or unconscious child what he or she will feel during the procedure. The family needs simple, direct explanations of their child's condition and proposed interventions. Parental presence should be guided by hospital policy, parents' coping abilities and staff's preference. If the family chooses to remain in the treatment room, a designated staff support person should remain with them to tend to their needs.

Nursing responsibilities are outlined in Table 6.11.

Table 6.11.   Nursing Responsibilities

NURSING ACTIONS	RATIONALE
1. Explain to the child and the family the need for the venous cutdown. Time may not allow for this preparation.	Enhances their understanding and cooperation.
2. Assemble the necessary equipment at the child's bedside. Assist with preparing the sterile field.	Perform as an aseptic procedure to prevent infection.
3. Don gloves and goggles.	Complies with universal precautions.
4. Assist the physician with selecting an appropriate site for the venous cutdown. The preferred site is the saphenous vein in the ankle.	
5. Immobilize on an arm board the extremity to be used for venous cutdown. Restrain the extremity manually or with a soft restraint.	Allows for safety and helps in maintaining a sterile field during catheter insertion.
6. Cleanse the skin with the povidone–iodine solution.	Prevents infection.
7. Assist the physician in anesthetizing the skin with a local anesthetic.	Decreases pain and discomfort during the procedure.
8. Assist the physician with venesection. Use sterile technique.	Venous cutdown is a physician's responsibility.
9. After cannulation, connect the catheter to the continuous IV infusion system. Assist the physician with suturing the catheter in place.	Allows for administration of fluids and medications; maintains a patent catheter.
10. Dress the site with a sterile dressing.	Aids in preventing infection.

Table 6.11.   (*cont.*)

NURSING ACTIONS	RATIONALE
11. Place a protective device over the site, and immobilize the extremity, as appropriate.	Prevents inadvertent dislodgment of the catheter.
12. Document the site of the catheter insertion, the size of the catheter, how the child tolerated the procedure, the estimated blood loss, and the type and rate of IV infusion.	Communicates the nursing interventions and observations to health-care professionals.

ASSISTING WITH CENTRAL VENOUS CANNULATION

Indications   Central venous access is indicated for fluid and medication administration to the central circulation, measurement of CVP, repeated venous blood sampling, and placement of a temporary pacemaker.

Contraindications   No absolute contraindications, although the procedure may be risky in children with bleeding tendencies.

Complications   Infection, hematoma, hemorrhage, thrombosis, pneumothorax, hemothorax, hydrothorax, cardiac tamponade, air embolism, and catheter fragment embolism.[1]

Equipment

> Venous catheters[1]
> > 21 gauge needle, 8 cm in length: infants < 1 year
> > 20 gauge needle, 12 cm in length: children 1–12 years
> > 18 gauge needle, 20 cm in length: children > 12 years
>
> Intracaths[1]
> > 22 gauge catheter with 19 gauge needle: infants < 1 year
> > 18 gauge catheter with 16 gauge needle: children 1–12 years
> > 16 gauge catheter with 14 gauge needle: children > 12 years
>
> Povidone–iodine solution
> 3-cc syringe with 25-gauge needle for local anesthetic
> Local anesthetic (1% or 2% lidocaine, per physician preference)
> Two 3-cc syringes (1 for flush and 1 discard sample)
> Normal saline (NS)
> Tape
> Soft restraints
> Blankets for positioning
> Suture material
> Sterile draping towels
> Sterile gloves
> Sterile 4 × 4 gauge
> Dressing materials: 2 × 2 sterile gauze and tape, or transparent dressing
> IV infusion setup (assembled)
> IV infusion pump (recommended)
> Goggles

Psychosocial Considerations   Explain to the awake or unconscious child what he or she will feel during the procedure. The family needs simple, direct explanations of their child's condition and proposed interventions. Parental presence should be guided by hospital policy, parents' coping abilities and staff's preference. If the family chooses to remain in the treatment room, a designated staff support person should remain with them to tend to their needs.

Nursing responsibilities are described in Table 6.12.

Table 6.12.   Nursing Responsibilities

NURSING ACTIONS	RATIONALE
1. Explain to the child and the family the need for central venous cannulation. Time may not allow for this preparation.	Enhances their understanding and cooperation.
2. Assemble the equipment at the child's bedside.	Allows for timely completion of the procedure.
3. Assist the physician with selecting an appropriate site. Common sites include external jugular (EJ), internal jugular (IJ), femoral vein, or subclavian vein.	
4. Place the child in an optimal position, and restrain or sedate the child.	Appropriate positioning assists with ease of insertion and minimizes complications.
a. **EJ:** Place the child in a 20–30° Trendelenburg position with head turned away from the side to be punctured.[1]	For EJ cannulation, the right side is preferred, as the apex of the right lung is lower than the left lung. Cannulation to the right atrium is more direct, and there is a decreased risk of damage to the thoracic duct.[14]
b. **IJ:** Place the child in a 20–45° Trendelenburg position, with the head turned away from the side to be accessed.[1] Place a towel roll under the shoulders, or hyperextend the neck.[1]	
c. **Subclavian vein:** Place the child in a 20–30° Trendelenburg position with the head turned away from the side to be punctured.	
d. **Femoral vein:** Restrain the leg, and keep it slightly externally rotated.[1]	
5. Don gloves and goggles.	Complies with universal precautions.
6. Assist the physician with the procedure.	
7. After successful venous cannulation, assist with suturing the catheter in place. Apply a sterile dressing. Flush the catheter with normal saline.	Prevent accidental dislodgment of the catheter; maintains catheter patency.

Table 6.12. (*cont.*)

NURSING ACTIONS	RATIONALE
8. Verify the placement with a chest x-ray.	Ensures that the catheter is in the correct position.
9. Auscultate breath sounds; verify x-ray findings. Initiate infusion of IV fluids and medications.	Verifies that no pneumothorax has occurred.
10. Document the site of the catheter insertion, the size of catheter, the child's response to the procedure, the type and rate of the fluids and medications administered.	Communicates the nursing interventions and observations to health-care professionals.

BLOOD PRODUCT ADMINISTRATION

Indications   Blood products are administered for hypovolemic shock, anemia, and thrombocytopenia. They can also be administered to improve the oxygen-carrying capacity of the blood[19] or for clotting-factor replacement (fresh-frozen plasma, cryoprecipitate).

Contraindications   Lack of consent to receive blood products (e.g., Jehovah's Witness).

Complications   Hemolytic and nonhemolytic transfusion reactions, infection, and complications of IV therapy.[20]

Equipment

> Blood product
> Blood filter/tubing
> Normal saline
> IV infusion pump/syringe pump
> Blood warmer, if indicated
> Gloves

Psychosocial Considerations   Older children, adolescents and their families may express concerns regarding the possible transmission of the HIV virus through blood or blood products. Answer their questions honestly and assist them to weigh the risks and benefits associated with receiving or not receiving the recommended therapy.

Nursing responsibilities are described in Table 6.13.

Table 6.13. Nursing Responsibilities

NURSING ACTIONS	RATIONALE
1. Explain to the child and the family the need for the blood product. Time may not allow for this preparation.	Enhances their understanding and cooperation.
2. Obtain written consent, as per hospital policy. Specific hospital policies and procedures should be reviewed	

Table 6.13. *(cont.)*

NURSING ACTIONS	RATIONALE
prior to initiating any transfusion, for product-specific information on dosing, rate of infusion, tubing, and filters.	
3. Review the physician's order. The order should include the blood product, any special processing (irradiated, washed), any premedication, the volume of blood product, and the transfusion rate.	Allows for safe administration. Volume or dosage of product depends on the type of blood product and the child's weight.[21] Premedication may be indicated for children with a history of febrile, nonhemolytic reactions.[20]
4. If appropriate, obtain the type and a cross-match.	Typing identifies ABO and Rh blood groupings and the presence of antibodies.[21] Cross-matching determines recipient and donor compatibility.[21]
5. Secure adequate IV access.	The larger the bore of the IV catheter, the more rapidly the transfusion is infused. Needles as small as 27 gauge may be used to administer whole blood at rates up to 100 cc/hr and packed cells up to 50 cc/hr without significant hemolysis.[22]
6. After obtaining the blood product from the blood bank, double-check the child's name (utilize the Emergency Department identification (ID) band), birthdate, hospital ID number, donor unit number, blood product, blood type, and product expiration date with a second registered nurse or a physician.	Allows for safe administration.[26]
7. Don clean gloves.	Complies with universal precautions.
8. Prime the blood product administration set.	All blood products should be filtered.[22,23] Gross clot (170–200 mm or micrometers) screen filters are usually adequate.[23] The infusion device allows for controlled accurate administration.[21,23] A breakdown of blood products can occur due to the age or viscosity of the product or mechanical factors, such as the filter, tubing, infusion pump/syringe, needle/catheter size, and rate of infusion.[23]
9. Assess the child's status, including vital signs.	Allows for a baseline assessment.

Table 6.13. (cont.)

NURSING ACTIONS	RATIONALE
10. Warm the blood for children receiving rapid or massive transfusions.	Prevents myocardial temperature from falling and inducing cardiac dysrhythmias.[19,21,23]
11. Initiate the transfusion slowly. The total transfusion time should not exceed 4 hours. Observe for signs of a hemolytic transfusion reaction; such signs may include fever, chills, chest pain, hypotension, and hemoglobinuria.[19] Consider the child's cardiorespiratory and hemodynamic status when determining the infusion rate.	Allows for assessment of any transfusion reaction. Infusing within 4 hours prevents bacterial growth and red cell hemolysis.[19] The infusion rate varies for differing blood components[21] and the child's health condition.
12. Stop the transfusion immediately if signs of a reaction are apparent. Notify the physician and the blood bank.	Transfusion reactions in neonates and children are difficult to categorize.[24] Most pediatric reactions are nonimmunological.[24]
13. Assess the child's status and vital signs every 30 minutes throughout the duration of the transfusion or more frequently as the child's condition warrants.	Allows for ongoing assessment for transfusion reaction, fluid overload, and IV infiltration.
14. If the transfusion is stopped, maintain IV access with the administration of NS.	Maintenance of a patent IV will allow for emergency drug and fluid administration.
15. If multiple units are transfused, monitor the child's serum potassium and calcium.	Potassium may increase if the blood product is stored, due to red cell breakdown.[19] Ionized calcium may decrease, as calcium binds with the citrate in the blood preservative.[19]
16. Don clean gloves to discontinue the transfusion.	Complies with universal precautions.
17. After the transfusion is complete, flush the IV with NS.	Clears the blood product from the IV line.
18. Document the blood product information (blood product type, number, signatures of the two registered nurses who checked the blood product), the vital signs obtained, and the child's response to the transfusion.	Communicates the nursing interventions and observations to health-care professionals.

MEDICAL ANTI-SHOCK TROUSER (MAST)
(Also known as the Pneumatic Antishock Garment—PASG)

Indications The MAST is indicated in the treatment of hypovolemic shock, with resultant hypotension, defined as systolic blood pressure less than one fourth to one third of normal for age.[32] Other indications include pelvic or lower-extremity fractures[25,26,27,28,29] and intra-abdominal hemorrhage. The MAST counteracts hypovolemia by application of counterpressure around the legs and abdomen, thus increasing systemic peripheral resistance.[26] The device also redistributes the blood flow from the periphery to the central circulation.[29]

Contraindications

Absolute Pulmonary edema or signs of pulmonary congestion;[25,26,27,29] inflation of the abdominal segment in pregnant women and in abdominal evisceration.[27]

Relative Isolated head injury;[27] cerebral edema;[25] impaled object in the abdomen or legs;[27] uncontrolled bleeding above the site of the MAST.[25,27]

Complications Compartment syndrome;[29] acidosis, decreased renal function, vomiting, respiratory compromise, trophic skin changes.[25]

Equipment

> Toddler-mast®: Children ages 2–4 years
> Pedi-mast®: Children 46–58 inches in height and 40–100 lbs. in weight
> Adult-mast®
> Downsizable MAST (adjusts from pediatric through adult sizes)
> Foot pump with tubing
> BP cuff/sphygmomanometer
> Gloves
> Stethoscope

Psychosocial Considerations Because the MAST is used for trauma care, the child is already frightened and fearful because of the other invasive procedures done to her or him. Explain to the child that the trousers are helping to keep his or her legs still and that she or he will be able to move their legs again after the trousers are removed.

The parents need to be told why the child has the MAST in place, as well as a brief explanation of how they work.

Nursing responsibilities are described in Tables 6.14 and 6.15.

Table 6.14. Nursing Responsibilities for the Inflation of Trousers

NURSING ACTIONS	RATIONALE
1. Explain to the child and the family the need for the MAST. Time may not allow for this preparation.	Enhances their understanding and cooperation.
2. Select the appropriate size of MAST; don gloves.	An appropriate size of garment extends from the edge of the rib margin to above the ankle.

Table 6.14.   (cont.)

NURSING ACTIONS	RATIONALE
3. Obtain the child's vital signs at least every 5 minutes, or more frequently, as the child's condition warrants.	Allows for ongoing hemodynamic assessment.
4. Open the garment and lay it flat.[26]	
5. Logroll the child and place the child supine on the garment.[27] Maintain the cervical spine alignment if cervical spine injury is suspected.	Prevents further injury.
6. The top of the garment should lie just below the lowest rib.[26]	Prevents potential respiratory compromise or impaired chest excursion.
7. Wrap the garment around the left leg and secure it with the Velcro® straps.[26]	Follows the proper sequence for the application process.
8. Wrap the garment around the right leg and secure it with the Velcro® straps.[26]	
9. Place the abdominal segment in the appropriate position, and secure it with the Velcro® straps.[26]	
10. Close the abdominal section valve, and inflate the leg sections using the foot pump.[26]	
11. Close the leg section valve, and open the abdominal section valve.[27]	
12. Inflate the abdominal section unless contraindicated.[27] Observe for respiratory distress with inflation of the abdominal compartment.	Inflate the abdominal section cautiously in children, as inflation of the abdominal compartment may decrease diaphragmatic excursion and may compromise respiratory effort.
13. Inflate the garment until air exhausts the pop-off valve, the child's BP stabilizes,[29] or the Velcro® straps stretch.	In each compartment, there is an automatic pressure release valve, so that pressure cannot exceed 104 mm Hg.[28]
14. Close the inflation/deflation valve when fully inflated.[26]	Allows for maintenance of pressure.
15. Auscultate breath sounds for pulmonary congestion.[27]	Fluid overload may occur.[28]
16. The MAST remains inflated until the child is hemodynamically stable.	
17. Document the time of inflation, the vital signs, and the child's response to the MAST application and inflation.*	Communicates the nursing interventions and observations to health-care professionals.

Table 6.15. Nursing Responsibilities for the Deflation of Trousers

NURSING ACTIONS	RATIONALE
1. Ensure that two large-bore IVs are in place and that fluid resuscitation has been initiated.	Premature removal of the trousers prior to treating hypovolemia may result in irreversible shock.[26]
2. Continue to obtain vital signs at frequent intervals.	
3. With the physician present, gradually deflate the abdominal compartment by opening the valve.	The abdominal compartment is deflated first, to prevent excessive pooling of blood in the lower extremities.[28]
4. Continue with deflation until a decrease in systolic BP of 5 mm Hg occurs.[26]	Slow deflation of the trousers allows for replacement of the circulating blood volume and restores circulation to poorly perfused body parts.[26]
5. Administer fluid replacement, as needed.	
6. When BP is stabilized, continue with gradual deflation of the right leg, then the left leg by opening the valves.	
7. Document the time of deflation, the vital signs, and the child's response to the MAST deflation.	Communicates the nursing interventions and observations to health-care professionals.
8. Wear gloves when removing the MAST from the child, as blood and body fluids may be present. Follow the manufacturer's instructions, for cleaning the MAST after its use.	Prevents contamination of self and others.

CARDIOPULMONARY RESUSCITATION (CPR)

The following section is based on recent American Heart Association recommendations for CPR in infants and children.[1] Table 6.16 summarizes CPR techniques in infants, children, and adults.

Indications   Closed cardiac massage is initiated to maintain oxygenation, ventilation, and circulation in the absence of spontaneous heartbeat and respirations.

Contraindications   None known.

Complications   Rib fractures, lung, liver, stomach injury.

Equipment

> 1 or 2 certified cardiopulmonary resuscitation (CPR) provider(s)
> Hard, flat surface (Cardiac board or short back board)
> Bag-valve-mask device
> Gloves

Psychosocial Considerations   When the child is in cardiac arrest, the family requires crisis intervention. See Chapter 2, Psychosocial Considerations for the Child and Family.

Nursing responsibilities are described in Table 6.17.

Table 6.16. Summary of CPR Techniques in Infants, Children, and Adults

	INFANT 0–1 YEAR	CHILD 1–8 YEARS	ADULT >8 YEARS
Initial breaths	2	2	2
Pulse check	Brachial	Carotid	Carotid
Correct hand placement for compression	2–3 fingers on lower third of sternum	Heel of one hand on lower third of sternum	Heel of both hands on lower sternum
Compression depth	$1/2$–1 inch 1.3–2.5 cm	1–$1^1/2$ inch 2.5–3.8 cm	$1^1/2$–2 inches 3.8–5 cm
Rate	100	80–100	80
Compression: ventilation ratio (one rescuer)	5:1	5:1	15:2
Compression: ventilation ratio (two rescuers)	5:1	5:1	5:1

Table 6.17. Nursing Responsibilities

NURSING ACTIONS	RATIONALE
1. Determine that the child is unresponsive, by gently shaking the infant or child. If unresponsive, continue with this sequence.	Vigorous attempts to arouse the infant or child should not be made, as they could cause further injury or worsen a spinal-cord injury.
2. Summon assistance immediately.	Allows for adequate support personnel.
3. Place the infant or child supine on a cardiac board or other hard surface.	Maximizes the effectiveness of external chest compressions.
4. Attempt to open the airway. a. Head-tilt/chin-lift: Using the hand closest to the child's head, tilt the head back into a neutral position for an infant or slightly hyperextend the head of a child. For the chin lift, place two fingers under the bony part of the lower jaw. (See Chapter 4.)	Moving the mandible forward may lift the tongue away from the airway.[25] With adequate jaw-muscle tone, lifting the head back will move the mandible forward and open the airway.[25] Jaw thrust is the safest airway positioning technique in cases where spinal cord injury is suspected.[1]

Table 6.17.   (*cont.*)

NURSING ACTIONS	RATIONALE
b. Jaw thrust: place two or three fingers on both sides of the lower jaw at the jaw angle, and lift upward. (See Chapter 4.)	
5. Look, listen, and feel for air exchange. If the child is not breathing, continue with this sequence.	
6. To breathe for the child, place a mask in the proper position, and seal the mouth. If a mask is not available, make a seal with your mouth over the mouth of a child or over the mouth and nose of an infant. (See Chapter 5.)	A tight seal allows for adequate ventilation.
7. Administer two breaths (1–1.5 seconds/breath) to the infant or child.	Breaths should produce adequate rise of the chest.[1] Administering breaths slowly aids in preventing gastric distention.
8. Assess for adequacy of circulation by palpating for the presence of a pulse. **a.** Infant—assess the brachial artery. **b.** Child—assess the carotid artery.	Absence of a pulse indicates ineffective or absent cardiac contractions. The carotid artery is accessible, as the neck area is easily exposed,[31] but the carotid artery may be difficult to palpate in infants, as their necks are short.[1]
9. If no pulse is present, begin cardiac compressions. **a.** *Infant:* Place the index finger of your hand closest to the feet one finger-breadth below the intermammary line (imaginary line drawn between the nipples). Compress the chest with two or three fingers (see Figure 6.8) to a depth of $1/2''$ to $1''$ at a rate of at least 100 times/minute.[31]	External chest compressions performed over the lower third of the sternum in infants and young children are more effective than midsternum compressions.[32]

Table 6.17. (*cont.*)

NURSING ACTIONS	RATIONALE

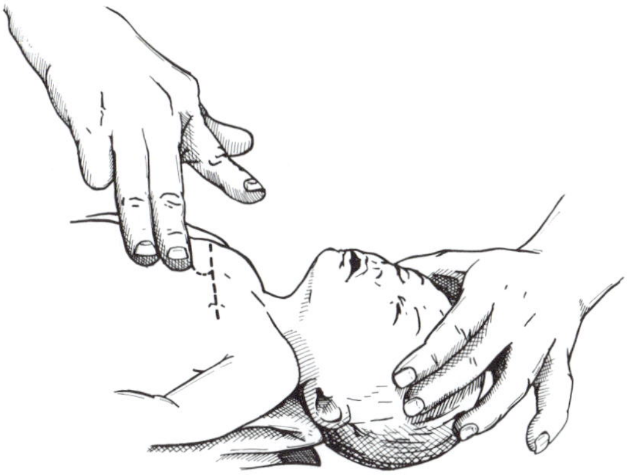

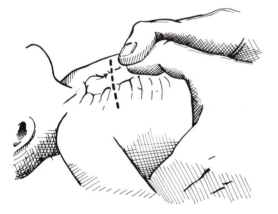

Figure 6.8. Proper finger placement for chest compressions in an infant. A folded towel helps to extend the neck and open the airway.

b. *Alternative position:* (i) Encircle the infant's chest with your hands, using your thumbs to compress the chest on the lower third of the sternum (see Figure 6.9a); (ii) compress to a depth of $^1/_2''$ to $1''$ at a rate of at least 100 times/minute.[31]

The alternative method may be used if a second rescuer is providing ventilatory support (see Figure 6.9b).

Figure 6.9. (a) Alternative method of hand placement for chest compressions in an infant.

c. *Child less than 8 years old:* Locate the correct hand position with the middle and index finger of

Table 6.17.   *(cont.)*

NURSING ACTIONS	RATIONALE

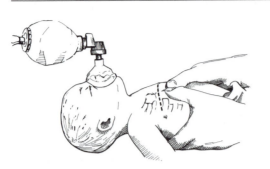

Figure 6.9.   **(b)** Basic life support measures in an infant. Note the slight hyperextension of the neck and the tight seal of the bag-valve mask device.

your hand closest to the child's feet. Trace with your fingers along the rib cage to the point where the ribs and the sternum meet. Place the heel of your opposite hand next to your index finger, with its heel parallel to the sternum. Compress the lower third of sternum to a depth of 1″ to 1¹/₂″ at a rate of 80–100 times/minute[31] (see Figure 6.10).

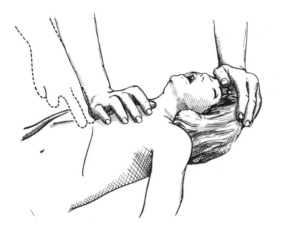

Figure 6.10.   Proper hand placement for chest compressions in a child. The fingers do not rest on the chest wall.

Table 6.17.   *(cont.)*

NURSING ACTIONS	RATIONALE
d. *Child older than 8 years* (up to an adult): Trace with your fingers along the rib cage to the point where the ribs and the sternum meet. Place the heel of your opposite hand next to the index finger (or two fingers if the child is adult size), with your heel parallel to the child's sternum. Place your second hand on top of your first. Compress the lower third of the sternum $1^1/_2''$ to $2''$, at a rate of 80 times/minute.[31]	Adult recommendations are used for children older than 8 years of age.[1]
10. Perform chest compressions while breathing for the child.[31]	For effective CPR, breathing and compressions must be coordinated.

a. One-rescuer CPR
    Infants: 5 compressions to 1 ventilation
    Child < 8 years: 5 compressions to 1 ventilation
    Child > 8 years: 15 compressions to 2 ventilations
    Reassess the child every 10 cycles.
	Count out loud to maintain a correct ratio.
	    Infant: "1-2-3-4-5-"
	    Child: "1-and-2-and-3-and-4-and-5-and-"

b. Two-rescuer CPR (all ages): 5 compressions to 1 ventilation.	
11. Initiate pediatric advanced life support, as the setting and the personnel allow. The Broselow Pediatric Resuscitation Tape allows for the rapid estimate of the child's weight based on height and recommends resuscitation medication dosages. See Figure 6.11.	*Advanced life support* is corrective-oriented, while *basic life support* is maintenance-oriented.

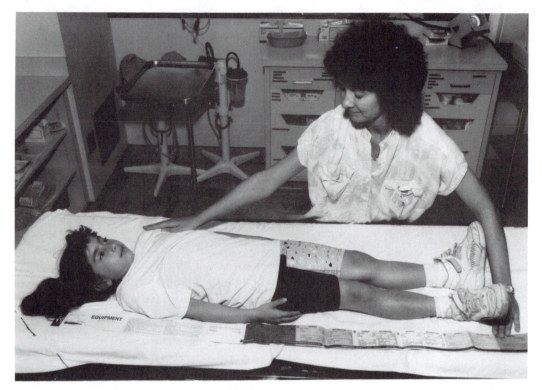

Figure 6.11. Use of the Broselow Pediatric Tape to calculate correct medication doses and proper resuscitative equipment sizes for children. (Tape courtesy of Broselow Medical Technologies)

Assisting with Defibrillation and Cardioversion

Indications   *Defibrillation* is used to interrupt disorganized electrical activity by using asynchronous direct current. *Cardioversion* is used to convert tachyarrythmias by using synchronized direct current.

Contraindications   Ventricular fibrillation not documented by ECG.

Complications   Adverse effects of electrical shock (burn).

Equipment

> ECG monitor and recorder
> Stethoscope
> BP cuff/sphygmomanometer
> Defibrillator
> External paddles:[1]
>   Infants: 4.5 cm diameter
>   Older children: 8.0 cm or 13 cm diameter
>   Adult: 14 cm diameter
> Conductive gel or cream
> Emergency cart and medications
> Airway equipment and oxygen

Psychosocial Considerations   Explain to the awake child prior to cardioversion that he or she will feel an electric shock or a jerk, if times allows. Administer IV sedation. The family needs simple, direct explanations of their child's condition and proposed interventions. Parental presence should be guided by hospital policy, parents' coping abilities and staff's preference. If the family chooses to remain in the treatment room, a designated staff support person should remain with them to tend to their needs.

Nursing responsibilities are described in Table 6.18.

Table 6.18. Nursing Responsibilities

NURSING ACTIONS	RATIONALE
1. Initiate basic life support; obtain emergency equipment and defibrillation.	Maintains minimal cardiac output to vital organs, in the absence of effective intrinsic cardiac output.
2. Verify ventricular fibrillation on ECG monitor. Assess for pulse/pulselessness. Consider sedation for the awake child during cardioversion.	Presence of ventricular fibrillation should be confirmed, as unnecessary treatment could prove harmful for the child.
3. Turn off an external pacemaker if in use.	Defibrillation may damage a pacemaker.
4. Select an appropriate paddle size. Paddle size should allow for good chest contact, with adequate separation to prevent bridging.	With bridging, the current will flow between the two paddles, across the chest surface rather than through the chest wall to the myocardium.[33]
5. Turn the defibrillator on. Select the synchronized mode for cardioversion.	Defibrillators are in asynchronous mode by default. The *asynchronous* mode is used for defibrillation. The *synchronous* mode is used for cardioversion of rhythms with distinguishable R waves.
6. Select the prescribed energy level on the defibrillator. Defibrillation: 2.0 Joules/kg. Cardioverson: 0.5–1.0 Joules/kg.	An optimal energy dose for children has not been established; controversy exists between the child's weight and energy dose.[1]
7. Apply the conductive gel or cream to the paddles; the prepackaged defibrillator pads may be too large for the child's chest.	A low-impedance medium is needed to reduce the resistance between the paddle and the skin.[1] Avoid saline-soaked pads, as conductivity is variable; alcohol pads can produce serious chest burns.[1]
8. Charge the defibrillator.	
9. Place the paddles on the chest.[1,25] a. One paddle is placed to the right of the upper sternum below the clavicle.	For effective defibrillation, the current must traverse the heart.[1]

Table 6.18.   *(cont.)*

NURSING ACTIONS	RATIONALE
b. The other paddle is placed below and to the left of the left nipple (see Figure 6.12).	For children with dentrocardia, a mirror image to a. and b. is used.

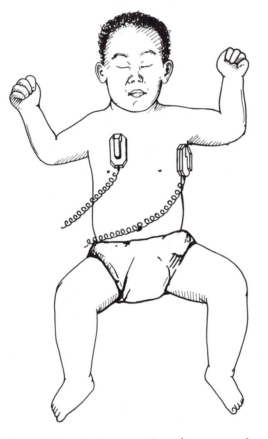

Figure 6.12. Proper anterior placement of defibrillator paddles (paddles not drawn to proportion).

c. Anterior–posterior position:[1,25] (1) One paddle is placed at the anterior precordial area; (2) the other paddle is placed at the posterior infrascapular area.	Often impractical during a resuscitation attempt.[1]
10. Apply firm pressure to the paddles.	
11. Clear the area. Make sure that assisting health-care professionals are not touching the child or the bed.	Reduces the risk of accidental shock.

Table 6.18.   *(cont.)*

NURSING ACTIONS	RATIONALE
12. Discharge the current.	
13. Recheck the rhythm and the presence of a pulse.	Provides data needed for determination of further intervention.
14. If ventricular fibrillation persists, double the energy level and defibrillate. Repeat defbrillation at the doubled energy level if necessary.[1] If cardioversion is unsuccessful, increase energy level to 2.0 Joules/kg.[1]	
15. Continue basic and advanced life support measures.	
16. If defibrillation or cardioversion is successful, monitor the child's ECG and vital signs, and treat precipitating factors.	In the postresuscitation period, close observation is essential to optimize the child's outcome.
17. Document the ECG strip pre- and postdefibrillation or cardioversion, the Joules/kg administered, and any medications administered.	Communicates the nursing interventions and observations to health-care professionals.

REFERENCES

1. Chameides L, ed. Textbook of pediatric advanced life support. Dallas, TX: American Academy of Pediatrics and American Heart Association, 1988:5, 7, 13–15, 37–40, 42–43, 66–67.
2. Hazinski MF. Nursing care of the critically ill child: A seven point check. Pediatr Nurs 1985;11:456–457.
3. *Idem.* Children are different. In: Hazinski MF, ed. Nursing care of the critically ill child. 2nd ed. St. Louis: C.V. Mosby, 1992:10.
4. Manley LK. Pediatric trauma: Initial assessment and management. J Emerg Nurs 1987;13:81.
5. Strange JM. Pediatric trauma. In: Strange JM, ed. Shock trauma care plans. Springhouse, PA: Springhouse Corp., 1987:305–306.
6. Curley MAQ. Pediatric cardiac dysrhythmias. Bowie, MD: Brady Communications Co., 1985:200–201.
7. Personal communication. Margaret C. Slota, R.N., M.N. November 21, 1990.
8. Task Force on Blood Pressure Control in Children. Report on the second task force on blood pressure control in children. Pediatrics 1987;79:3–4.
9. Moss AJ. Indirect methods of blood pressure measurement. Pediatr Clin North Am 1978;25:9, 13.
10. Miller KM. Venipuncture. In: Millar S, Sampson SK, Soukup SM, eds. AACN procedure manual for critical care. 2nd ed. Philadelphia: W.B. Saunders, 1985:42–44, 46.

11. Hodge D. Intraosseous infusions: A review. Pediatr Emerg Care, 1985; 1:216–217.

12. Glaeser PW, Losek JD, Nelson DB, et al. Pediatric intraosseous infusions: Impact on vascular access time. Am J Emerg Med 1988;6:330–332.

13. Manley L, Hale K, Dick M. Intraosseous infusion: A rapid vascular access for critically ill or injured infants and children. J Emerg Nurs 1988;14:65.

14. Pratt JL. Intraosseous infusion. Internat Pediatr 1989;4:20.

15. Peck KR, Altieri M. Intraosseous infusions: An old technique with modern applications. Pediatr Nurs 1988;14:296–297.

16. Lawless S, Orr R. Axillary arterial monitoring for pediatric patients. Pediatrics 1989;84:273.

17. DeGroot KD, Damato MB. Monitoring intra-arterial pressure. Crit Care Nurs 1986;6:75, 78.

18. Wetmore NE. Nursing responsibilities with arterial access. National Intravenous Therapy Association, 1981;4:429.

19. Davis JL. Blood administration. In: Kinkade SL, Lohrman J, eds. Critical care nursing procedures: A team approach. Philadelphia: B.C. Decker, 1990: 305–308, 310.

20. Freeman S, Haisfield ME, McGuire DB, Morell L, Paulaitis L, Wohlganger J. Nursing considerations in the administration of blood component therapy. Sem Oncol Nurs 1990;6:155–156.

21. Landier WC, Barrel ML, Styffe EJ. How to administer blood components to children. Am J Matern Child Nurs 1987;12:178–179, 182, 184.

22. Herrera AJ, Corless J. Blood transfusions: Effect of speed of infusion and of needle gauge on hemolysis. J Pediatr 1981;99:758.

23. Butch SH, Coltra MA. Techniques of transfusion. In: Kasprisin DO, Luban NL, eds. Pediatric transfusion medicine, Vol. 1. Boca Raton, FL: CRC Press, 1987:108–109, 111–112.

24. Luban NL. Adverse reactions to blood and blood products. In: Kasprisin DO, Luban NL, eds. Pediatric transfusion medicine, Vol. 2. Boca Raton, FL: CRC Press, 1987:128.

25. Schleien CL, Rogers MC. Cardiopulmonary resuscitation in infants and children. In: Rogers MC, ed. Textbook of pediatric intensive care. Baltimore: Williams & Wilkins, 1987:10, 30, 46–47.

26. Medical Anti-Shock Trousers (MAST). Product information booklet. David Clark Company, Inc., 360 Franklin St., Worcester, MA 01604. 5, 8–10.

27. Canan PJ. The pneumatic antishock garment. In: Strange JM, ed. Shock trauma care plans. Springhouse, PA: Springhouse Corp., 1987:340–341.

28. Slavik ME. Circulatory assist techniques. In: Persons CB, ed. Critical care procedures and protocols: A nursing process approach. Philadelphia: J.B. Lippincott, 1987:108, 111.

29. Ford PJ, Vislusky FM. External counterpressure with MAST garment. In: Millar S, Sampson LK, Soukup SM, eds. AACN procedure manual for critical care. 2nd ed. Philadelphia: W.B. Saunders, 1985:127–130.

30. Kaplan BH, Soderstrom CA. Pneumatic antishock garments and the compartment syndrome. Am J Emerg Med 1987;5:177–178.

31. Albarran-Sotelo R, Flint LS, Kelley KJ, eds. Instructor's manual for basic life support. Dallas: American Heart Association, 1987; 43, 66–68.

32. Orlowski JP. Optimum position for external cardiac compression in infants and children. Ann Emerg Med 1986;15:667.

33. Webster HW. Bioinstrumentation: Principles and techniques. In: Hazinski MF, ed. Nursing care of the critically ill child. 2nd ed. St. Louis: C.V. Mosby, 1992:983.

CHAPTER

7

Procedures Involving the Gastrointestinal and Genitourinary Systems

Bonnie Clemence

OVERVIEW OF PEDIATRIC GASTROINTESTINAL AND GENITOURINARY DIFFERENCES

The gastrointestinal (GI) tract has limited functioning until the child is 2–3 years of age, at which time it functions at the adult level.[1] Sucking and swallowing are present at birth, but swallowing is a reflexive action until 3 months of age. After the age of 6 months, the infant can voluntarily spit and swallow or retain food in her or his mouth. Complete differentiation of what tastes "good" or "bad" does not occur until the age of 6 years, which is why ingestions are common in the toddler and preschool age groups.

During the first 3–4 years of life, the abdominal musculature is weak, the abdominal organs are large, and the lower spine is lordotic, all of which produce a soft, protuberant belly.[2] These factors leave the abdominal organs susceptible to injury from blunt trauma. The bladder is an abdominal organ in the young child, and the kidneys are immature at birth. The glomerular filtration rate does not approximate adult values until the third year of life.[3]

Children who wear diapers are prone to urinary tract infections; girls are prone to vaginitis. Children achieve a regular pattern of bowel elimination by the preschool years and achieve nighttime urinary control by age 5 years.[4]

Reproductive anatomical differentiation occurs prior to birth and again during puberty. Both males and females are born with a complete reproductive system; however, many of its parts do not mature or begin to function until puberty.

ORAL HYDRATION

Indications   Oral hydration is indicated to prevent or treat dehydration in children. Rehydration with liquids is necessary to replace the water and electrolyte losses that occur with vomiting and diarrhea.

Contraindications   Greater than 5% decrease of body weight, an abnormal sodium level, and a blood urea nitrogen (BUN) greater than 25 mg/dL;[5] and inability to take and retain oral fluids.[5]

Complications   Hypo- or hypernatremia may result if an inappropriate oral solution is given.

Choice of Solutions   Clear liquids

> Infants[5] — Pedialyte™ or Lytren™
> Older children
>> Flat ginger ale or cola (can be made flat by adding a teaspoon of sugar and a teaspoon of water to 6–8 ounces of ginger ale or cola)
> Koolaid®
> Gatorade®
> Popsicles

Psychosocial Interventions   Encouraging an ill child to drink requires patience. Thirsty infants will wet their lips, suck on their hands, and try to put objects to their mouths. To facilitate swallowing, hold the infant in an upright position. Toddlers, due to their sense of autonomy, may refuse liquids even if they are thirsty. To encourage hydration, give them medicine cups with their choice of appropriate fluids, rather than asking them whether they want to drink. Popsicles are ideal for toddlers and preschoolers, as they can feed themselves and achieve autonomy.

The parents are understandably anxious about their child's vomiting and diarrhea. They may feel guilty for not bringing the child into the Emergency Department sooner or may feel inadequate because their child is unable to take and retain fluids. When assisting the child to drink, families need emotional support to cope with their own anxieties so that they will not convey their anxieties to the child. Constant reassurance with the parents is beneficial to promoting a calm parent–child interaction.

Nursing responsibilities are described in Table 7.1.

Table 7.1. Nursing Responsibilities

NURSING ACTIONS	RATIONALE
1. Obtain the nude weight of the infant. In a child over 2 years of age, weigh the child with underwear only.	Provides a baseline for ongoing assessments.
2. Obtain a history from the parent, including the number of stools and their consistency, the number of emeses, the number of wet diapers in the past 24 hours, the time of the last wet diaper or when child last voided. Observe the child's mucous	The time of the last known urinary output may be indicative of the extent of dehydration.

Table 7.1. *(cont.)*

NURSING ACTIONS	RATIONALE
membranes, level of activity, and skin turgor. In crying infants and young children, observe for tearing. If the child has urinated, obtain a urine-specific gravity (should be < 1.020), and check for the presence of ketones.	
3. Explain to the child and the family the need for the hydration. Ask how the child usually drinks fluids (bottle, cup, etc.). Offer options, and ask the child about fluid preference.	Enhances their understanding and cooperation. Also provides the parents with the necessary knowledge to carry out the procedure.
4. If the child has been vomiting, begin with 5 to 15 milliliters by spoon or medicine cup every 10 to 15 minutes.[6] If vomiting occurs, wait 20 minutes and restart with 5 to 10 milliliters of fluid.[6]	Small amounts keep the stomach from becoming overdistended, thereby preventing further irritation.
5. If 1 tablespoon is retained, increase the amounts to 1 ounce every $1/2$ hour for 2 hours, slowly increasing the amount of liquid and the time between administrations.	Gradual amounts slowly acclimate the stomach to fluids and increases the likelihood of fluid retention.
6. Continue with clear liquids for 24 hours, then introduce a diet, as follows: Breast-fed infants—resume breast feeding. Other infants under 1 year: clear fluids for 24 hours, then half-strength formula gradually increased to full-strength formula over a day or two.[6] Children over 1 year, advance to light diet (see the BRAT diet, described in Step 8), then increase to regular diet.	The gradual introduction of foods prevents the recurrence of vomiting.
7. If the primary problem is diarrhea, children can usually tolerate larger volumes of fluids than with vomiting.	
8. With diarrhea, for children older than 1 year—continue clear liquids for 12–24 hours. Begin bananas, rice cereal, applesauce, and toast or crackers (BRAT diet). This diet should be continued for 48–72 hours before returning to a regular diet.	These foods tend to make the bowel movements firm.

Table 7.1. (*cont.*)

NURSING ACTIONS	RATIONALE
9. Assess the child for further vomiting and/or diarrhea. If vomiting or diarrhea continues, IV rehydration may be necessary (see the procedure on IV therapy, in Chapter 6).	Continual assessment provides the nurse with data to decide when to initiate other measures.
10. Document how well the child tolerated oral hydration, as well as vital signs, urinary output, further episodes of vomiting and/or diarrhea, level of activity, and the amount and kind of fluid retained. Document the instructions given to the parents.	Communicates the nursing interventions and observations to health-care professionals.

NASOGASTRIC TUBE PLACEMENT

Indications   A nasogastric (NG) tube is inserted to decompress the stomach and the proximal bowel, in response to obstruction or trauma; for gastric lavage, in the presence of upper GI bleeding or ingestion; and for the administration of medications and nutrition.[8]

Contraindications   Presence of major facial, head or spinal trauma;[10] in these circumstances, the oropharyngeal route is preferred.

Complications   Tracheal intubation, nasal trauma, vomiting (leading to aspiration),[8] passage into the cranium in the presence of basilar skull fractures.

Preparation of Equipment

> NG tube of the correct size
>> Newborn/Infant—size 8 French
>> Toddler/preschooler size 10 French
>> School age size 12 French
>> Adolescent size 14–16 French
> Catheter-tip syringe
> Emesis basin
> Water soluble lubricant
> Tape (adhesive or waterproof)
> Stethoscope
> Suction device
> Suction catheters
> Gloves, goggles, mask, gown if needed

Psychosocial Considerations   While NG-tube insertion is not a difficult or painful procedure, it is very anxiety producing for the child. Infants and young children do not like having their heads held still or their faces touched under normal circumstances, let alone during an intrusive procedure. Allow them to move another part of their bodies (i.e., fingers, feet, toes). The older child can participate in the procedure by holding the tape, syringe, and so forth; this participation gives the child a sense of control. If time permits, demonstrating the procedure on a doll may be helpful. Telling children to take slow, deep breaths and to swallow during the procedure also gives them a sense of control and serves as a distraction while allowing the tube to be passed easily.

Do not ask the parents to hold the child's head during the procedure. The child can easily believe he or she has been betrayed by the parent, which will cause more distress for both the parent and the child. Allow the parent to hold and comfort the child as soon as possible after the NG tube has been inserted. Always praise the child for cooperating, as this gives the child a sense of mastery.

Nursing responsibilities are described in Table 7.2.

Table 7.2.   Nursing Responsibilities

NURSING ACTIONS	RATIONALE
1. Explain to the child and the family the need for NG tube insertion. Reassure the child that the NG tube will help her or his stomach to feel better. Obtain the assistance of additional personnel before beginning the procedure.	Enhances their understanding and cooperation. Assures proper readiness of child.
2. Measure the nasogastric tube by placing the distal end of the tube at the tip of the nose and extending it to the earlobe and down to the xiphoid process (see Figure 7.1). Mark the estimated length of the NG tube, using a piece of tape.	Measurement of the nasogastric tube before insertion provides a better estimate of placement into the stomach.
3. Have the suction device turned on, with the appropriate catheter attached, to assist in removal of secretions/vomitus.	Ensures preparation in case of aspiration or choking during the NG-tube insertion.
4. Position the child for NG-tube insertion	
a. Place infants and unresponsive children supine, with their head turned toward the side.[8] Ensure airway patency prior to tube insertion.	Allows for easy passage of the tube and prevents obstruction of the airway; prevents aspiration.
b. Place an awake, cooperative child in a high Fowler's position, with head slightly flexed.	
5. Don gloves; use goggles, mask, and gown if needed.	Complies with universal precautions.
6. Place the water-soluble lubricant on the distal end of the tube.	Prevents irritation to nasal passage and increases the ease of insertion.
7. Encourage the awake child to swallow or sip water or to flex her or his head (if permitted) during tube insertion; flex the infant's neck, if needed.[9]	Facilitates passage of the tube and assists with glottic closure.[8]

Table 7.2.   (*cont.*)

NURSING ACTIONS	RATIONALE

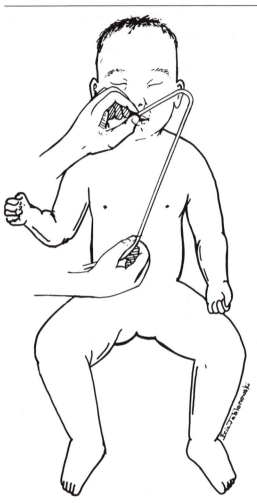

Figure 7.1.   Measurement of a nasogastric tube prior to insertion.

8. Insert the tube through the naris, directing it straight back, not upward, along the floor of the nose.[8] Do not force the tube if an obstruction is met.	Facilitates passage of the tube through the nasopharynx.
9. Insert the tube to the measured length. If the child develops signs of respiratory distress or is unable to cry or to speak, promptly remove the tube and attempt reinsertion.	Allows for ease of insertion; prevents aspiration or trauma.
10. Check for the correct NG tube placement by introducing 10 cc of air into the tube, using the catheter-tip sy-	Ensures proper placement.

Table 7.2.   (*cont.*)

NURSING ACTIONS	RATIONALE
ringe, while listening over the stomach with the stethoscope for a popping sound of air. Aspirate approximately 10 cc of gastric contents into the syringe.	
11. Tape the tube into place. Apply benzoin on the child's upper lip (and cheek for infants or toddlers) to keep the tube secure (see Figure 7.2).	Prevents movement of tube from the measured position.

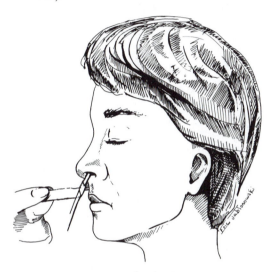

Figure 7.2. One method of taping a nasogastric tube. Benzoin may be applied to the upper lip before taping. Additional reinforcement may be accomplished in infants and small children by taping a loop of the tube to the cheek.

12. Give the child something to hold after the procedure is completed (a toy or security blanket).	The child may attempt to remove the NG tube; giving the child something to hold serves as a distraction from the NG tube.
13. Praise the child for cooperating during the procedure.	
14. Document the time of insertion, the tube size, the amount and characteristics of the gastric contents, and how the child tolerated the procedure. Document the results of a guiac test, if performed.	Communicates the nursing interventions and observations to health-care professionals.

GASTRIC LAVAGE

Indications   Gastric lavage is indicated to empty the stomach in toxic ingestions and to control upper GI bleeding. It is used in children with an altered level of consciousness, when emesis is not preferred.

Contraindications   Caustic ingestions and in most hydrocarbon ingestions.

Complications   Aspiration (especially if obtunded/comatose child is not endotracheally intubated prior to lavage).

Preparation of Equipment

> Nasogastric tube
> > Infants and young children: 12 French
> > Older children and adolescents: 24 French (up to 36 French)[10]
> Oropharyngeal tube (50 orogastric)[10]
> Normal saline or 0.45 (45 percent) normal saline solution[10]
> Catheter-tip syringe
> Oxygen; suction device and suction catheter
> Emesis basins
> Water soluble lubricant
> Stethoscope
> Gloves; goggles, mask and gown if needed

Psychosocial Considerations   As with NG-tube insertion, this procedure is not well tolerated in the awake and active child. Explain to the awake or unconscious child what he or she will feel (i.e., "fullness in your tummy"). Give older children a simple explanation of what is happening, as they have a better understanding of their bodies' structure and function. Provide distraction, such as taking deep breaths.

Usually, gastric lavage is needed as an emergency intervention with poisonings and bleedings. Therefore, the family may already be distressed because of the circumstances necessitating the emergency department visit. The parents should not restrain the child for this procedure; if the parents desire to be present, have them talk with the child and help the child with deep-breathing exercises. These actions allow the parents to help their child during the procedure.

Nursing responsibilities are described in Table 7.3.

ASSISTING WITH PERITONEAL LAVAGE

Indications   Peritoneal lavage is a diagnostic procedure used to detect hemoperitoneum in children who have sustained multiple trauma and have evidence of abdominal signs or symptoms, altered sensorium, unexplained shock, or major thoracic or multisystem injuries.[11] As a rule, it is less useful in children than in adults and, thus, is often omitted in favor of an abdominal computed tomography (CT) scan.

Contraindications   A history of multiple abdominal operations, penetrating wounds of the abdomen, pregnancy or radiographic evidence of free air in the abdomen.

Table 7.3. Nursing Responsibilities

NURSING ACTIONS	RATIONALE
1. Ensure proper placement of the largest size of oropharyngeal or NG tube (see the preceding procedure on NG-tube placement). Don gloves; use goggles, mask and gown if needed.	Complies with universal precautions.
2. Position the child on her or his left side, with the head slightly lower than the feet.[10] Or, position the child upright.	
3. Aspirate the stomach contents; send the specimen to the laboratory for analysis, if indicated. Perform a guiac test, if indicated.	Provides identification of any toxic substances; identifies presence of blood.
4. Connect the catheter-tip syringe to the gastric tube, and instill (a) 50–100 cc of 0.45 (45%) or normal saline in young children, or (b) 150–200 cc of 0.45 normal saline in adolescents.[10]	Slow instillation prevents vomiting and possible aspiration.
5. Slowly aspirate the solution from the gastric tube, using a syringe or a suction device.	Provides an accurate measure of amounts instilled and aspirated.
6. Repeat Steps 2 and 3 until the solution is clear, using approximately 500–1000 cc in infants and young children, and at least 2000 cc in adolescents.[10] Ensure that all saline instilled is removed. Prepare the child for removal of the gastric tube, by securing her or him, as needed.	Ensures removal of toxic substances.
7. Remove the gastric tube slowly, if indicated.	
8. Praise the child for cooperating and make her or him comfortable.	
9. Document the time, the size of the gastric tube, the type and amount of the instilled solution, the characteristics and amount of the gastric contents, and how the child tolerated the procedure. If the gastric contents were sent for analysis, document the time when sent and the time when results were obtained.	Communicates the nursing interventions and observations to health-care professionals.

Complications   Peritonitis; perforation of the abdominal viscera; hemorrhage; false-positive results that are due to bleeding from the incision or blunt trauma to the bowel;[8] leakage of the peritoneal fluid.

Preparation of Equipment

> Cutdown tray
> Povidone–iodine solution
> Peritoneal catheter
> Local anesthetic: 1% lidocaine with epinephrine
> 25 gauge 1$^{1}/_{2}$″ needle
> 5-cc syringe
> 1 L warmed lactated Ringer's solution
> 10-cc syringe
> IV tubing—maxidrip solution set
> Scalpel blade (#15) and handle
> Sterile drapes
> Suture material
> Sterile 4 × 4 gauze pads
> Gloves, goggles, mask and gown, if needed

Psychosocial Considerations   This procedure occurs whenever other invasive procedures have been performed (venipuncture, catheterization, etc.). Explain to the awake or unconscious child what the insertion and the fluid will feel like. If the child is awake, have the parent or another nurse help with deep breathing exercises or hold the child's hands.

Nursing responsibilities are described in Table 7.4.

Table 7.4.   Nursing Responsibilities

NURSING ACTIONS	RATIONALE
1. Explain to the child and the family the need for the peritoneal lavage. Time may not permit this preparation. Seek assistance from additional personnel prior to beginning procedure.	Enhances their understanding and cooperation. Assists with ease of completing the procedure.
2. Pass an NG tube, to decompress the stomach, and a urinary catheter, to empty the bladder.[8]	
3. Don sterile gloves, and cleanse the site with povidone–iodine solution, and drape with a sterile towel.	Decreases the risk of contamination.
4. The physician injects a local anesthetic.	Prevents discomfort from incision and catheter insertion.
5. The physician makes an incision approximately 1–2 cm above the umbilicus.[8]	The midline area of the abdomen is relatively avascular. A supraumbilical location is preferable in younger children, whose bladders extend into their abdomens.

Table 7.4. (*cont.*)

NURSING ACTIONS	RATIONALE
6. The physician inserts the catheter into the peritoneal cavity.	
7. The physician attaches a 10-cc syringe to the catheter and aspirates the peritoneal contents.	
8. If no blood is aspirated, attach IV tubing to 1 L of warmed lactated Ringer's solution and infuse at 10–20 cc/kg.[8]	Warmed solution promotes comfort and prevents abdominal pain. Infusion of 10 cc/kg prevents overdistention of the abdomen.
9. Turn the child from side to side if the child's condition permits.[8]	Promotes distribution of the solution throughout the peritoneal cavity.[8]
10. Lower the IV bag, and allow the fluid to return by gravity.	Effluent should be returned within 5–10 minutes. Repositioning of the child may facilitate drainage.
11. Send approximately 30 cc of peritoneal fluid to the laboratory for analysis. Specimens should be sent for:[9] Complete blood count Amylase level Gram stain Bile Culture	Laboratory analysis is required to provide definitive diagnosis.
12. Lavage is considered positive if any of the following are present:[9] Grossly bloody or blood-tinged fluid Red blood count (RBC) > 100,000 red blood cells (rbc)/mm^3 White blood count (WBC) > 500 white blood cells (wbc)/cc Presence of stool	
13. The physician removes the catheter and sutures the wound. Apply a sterile dressing.	Prevents further contamination of peritoneal cavity.
14. Document the time, the type of catheter, the amount and type of solution instilled, the character of the returned solution, the results obtained from laboratory analysis, the wound closure and dressing, and how the child tolerated the procedure.	Communicates the nursing interventions and observations to health-care professionals.

URINE BAG APPLICATION

Indications   A urine bag is used in young children (under 2 years) and for children who are not toilet trained, to collect a urine specimen for laboratory analysis. A urine bag is also indicated to collect urine for measurement of intake and output.

Contraindications   A urine bag should not be placed on a child with excoriated skin from a diaper rash. If a sterile specimen is needed for culture, collecting urine from a bag may not be advisable.

Complications   Irritation to the skin from the adhesive on the urine bag.

Preparation of Equipment

> Urine collection bag (newborn or pediatric)
> Washcloths (at least 3) or nonsterile 4 × 4 gauze pads
> Mild soap
> Clean diaper
> Gloves

Psychosocial Considerations   Removing the bag is probably more uncomfortable than placing it on the child. Encourage parents to comfort and distract the child while the bag is applied or removed.

> Nursing responsibilities are described in Table 7.5.

ASSISTING WITH SUPRAPUBIC ASPIRATION (BLADDER TAP)

Indications   Suprapubic aspiration (bladder tap) is a method of obtaining a sterile urine specimen in an infant or child less than 2 years of age.[8]

Contraindications   The aspiration should not be attempted in the infant or child who has recently voided. It is best to wait at least 1 hour after voiding before attempting the procedure.[8]

Complications   Bleeding from puncture site,[1] hematuria,[1,8] bowel perforation.[8]

Preparation of Equipment

> Sterile 3-cc syringe
> Sterile 20-, 21-, or 22-gauge 1-inch needle
> Sterile 22-gauge 1¹/₂-inch spinal needle
> Alcohol wipes
> Povidone–iodine wipes
> Sterile 2 × 2 gauze pads
> Sterile specimen container
> Clean diaper
> Band-Aid™
> Gloves

Psychosocial Considerations   This procedure requires the infant to remain very still; however, the infant should be allowed to move his or her hands or

Table 7.5. Nursing Responsibilities

NURSING ACTIONS	RATIONALE
1. Explain to the child and the family the need for the urine bag.	Enhances their understanding and cooperation.
2. Remove the child's diaper.	Exposes the area where bag will be applied.
3. Wet one cloth, and place a small amount of soap on it. Wet another cloth with plain water.	Prepares for cleansing of diaper area.
4. Cleanse the genital area (see Table 7.7).	Ensures that the bag will adhere properly. A bag will not adhere to skin that is oily, moist, or powdered.
5. Dry the diaper area thoroughly with a third cloth. Remove the backing from the bag, exposing the adhesive.	Enhances bag application.
6. Position the child.	Promotes ease in application.
a. *Female* — Place the child in a supine frogleg position. Place the bag at the upper part of the vulva, and secure it to the perineum, or place one side of the bag on first, then the other side.	
b. *Male* — Place the child in a supine position. Place the penis inside the bag.	
7. Ensure that the adhesive is attached firmly to the genital area.	Avoids leakage.
8. Apply a dry diaper after the bag is applied.	Promotes comfort.
9. Check the bag frequently; remove when urine is obtained.	Prevents skin irritation.
10. Document the time of bag application; note the amount, color, and odor of the specimen. Note any skin irritation.	Communicates the nursing interventions and observations to health-care professionals.

head. Offer the infant a pacifier during the procedure. The older infant can hold onto a security object. Due to the infant's larger ratio of body surface area to weight, keep the room warm. Warm your hands before positioning the child, to increase comfort and decrease distress.

Offer the parents a choice to remain with the child or to remove themselves until the procedure is completed. If the family remains in the room, have them hold the child's hands and talk quietly to the child.

Nursing responsibilities are described in Table 7.6.

Table 7.6. Nursing Responsibilities

NURSING ACTIONS	RATIONALE
1. Explain to the parent the need for the bladder tap. Talk softly, and maintain eye contact with the infant.	Promotes parental understanding. Promotes the child's comfort.
2. Remove the diaper.	Exposes the area where the procedure is to be performed.
3. Place a urine collection bag for sterile urine culture (refer to Table 7.5).	Infants often void during bladder taps; this will help to obtain a urine specimen.
4. Place the child in a supine position, with arms securely restrained and legs held in the frogleg position.[8]	Prevents the child from moving during the procedure.
5. Clean the area above the symphysis pubis twice with povidone–iodine; allow the area to dry for a few seconds.	Prevents bacterial contamination.
6. Remove povidone–iodine with alcohol wipes.	
7. Attach the needle to 3-cc syringe, using sterile technique.	
8. The physician inserts the needle into the bladder, approximately 1 cm above the pubic bone and perpendicular to the skin (see Figure 7.3).	Allows for entry into the bladder.

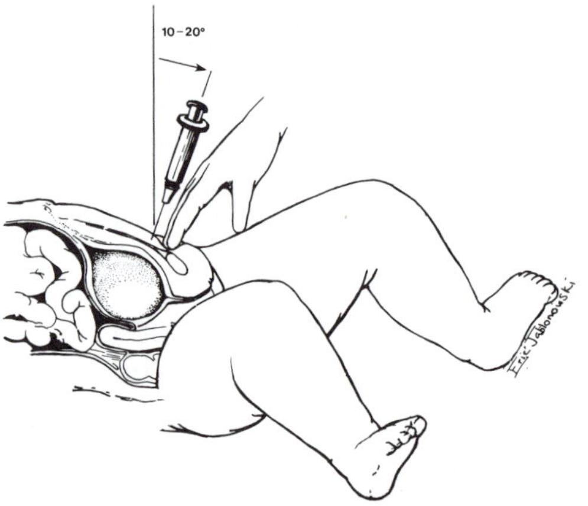

Figure 7.3. Proper placement of the syringe and needle for suprapubic aspiration.

9. The physician applies negative pressure to the syringe until urine is aspirated.	Collects urine sample.
10. The physician withdraws the needle.	

Table 7.6.   (*cont.*)

NURSING ACTIONS	RATIONALE
11. Hold pressure over the site with a 2 × 2 pad for 1–2 minutes. Apply a bandage.	Prevents bleeding at the site.
12. Apply a dry diaper, and comfort the infant.	Bladder may have spasms afterward.
13. Replace the needle with a syringe cap, or transfer the specimen to a sterile container.	Prevents contamination.
14. Send the specimen to laboratory for analysis. The specimen can be divided for urinalysis and culture.	Provides analysis of the urine content.
15. Document the needle size, the amount of urine obtained, the characteristics of the urine, whether bleeding occurred, and how the infant tolerated the procedure.	Communicates the nursing interventions and observations to health-care professionals.

BLADDER CATHETERIZATION

Indications   Bladder catheterization is performed to relieve urinary retention, to measure urinary output in critically ill or injured children, and to obtain a urine specimen for analysis.[11]

Contraindications   Evidence of blood at the urethral meatus;[11] perineal hematoma;[11] or urethral trauma.[8]

Complications   Urinary tract infection, vaginal catheterization, urethral and bladder trauma,[8] conversion of a partial urethral tear to a complete tear.[11]

Preparation of Equipment

> Sterile catheterization kit
> Urinary catheters[12]
>> Newborn — 5–8 French feeding tube
>> 6 months to one year — 5–8 French catheter
>> 1–3 years — 10 French catheter
>> 4–7 years — 10–12 French catheter
>> 8–10 years — 12 French catheter

Psychosocial Considerations   Toddlers and preschoolers can easily misinterpret the rationale for the procedure, due to their heightened interest in and fantasies about their private parts. They may view this procedure as punishment for bedwetting or for masturbation. School-age children and adolescents are modest about their bodies. They need clear and simple explanations of what is being done and why. Encourage them to take deep breaths to facilitate the passage of the catheter and to lessen their anxiety. Tell both younger and older children what sensations they may experience, such as cold soap, pressure in their private parts, and a feeling of urinary urgency. Ask the parents which word the child uses for urination. Children need to be told that they are permitted to urinate once the catheter is in, as they may have fears that they will wet the bed.

Again, parents should be given the choice of staying or leaving during the procedure. Respect the child's need for privacy if he or she wishes the parent to leave. If the child is of the opposite sex of the nurse, it may be necessary to have a second nurse present. Try to have a nurse of the same sex perform the procedure if at all possible. Never have the family restrain the child during catheterization because of the sense of betrayal the child may experience. Encourage the parent to comfort the child immediately after the procedure. If the catheter is going to be indwelling, remind the child that they will not wet the bed and give her or him permission to urinate. Allow the child to hold onto her or his transitional object or a favorite toy to distract the child and prevent the child's removal of the indwelling catheter.

Nursing responsibilities are described in Table 7.7.

Table 7.7. Nursing Responsibilities

NURSING ACTIONS	RATIONALE
1. Explain to the child and the family the need for the catheterization.	Enhances their understanding and cooperation.
2. Seek assistance from additional personnel prior to beginning the procedure.	Ensures proper positioning of child to avoid urethral injury.
3. Ensure adequate lighting.	Assists in identifying the meatus (especially in females).
4. Place a sterile catheter tray near the meatus. Open the tray, using sterile technique.	Tray covering can be used as a sterile field.
5. Put on sterile gloves, and arrange the equipment in order of its use. If an indwelling Foley catheter is used, test the balloon by inflating it; check for leaks, and deflate the balloon.	Increases efficiency; detects possible leak or defect in the balloon prior to insertion.
6. Arrange drapes around the meatal opening.	Increases size of sterile field.
7. Lubricate the end of the catheter with a water-soluble lubricant.	Lubrication reduces friction and facilitates catheter insertion.
8. Cleanse the area, using povidone–iodine wipes (or cotton balls saturated with povidone–iodine).	Reduces introduction of microorganisms into bladder.
9. Position the child. a. *For females*—Place the child in	Promotes visualization of the meatus.

Table 7.7.   (*cont.*)

NURSING ACTIONS	RATIONALE
the frogleg position. Separate the labia minora with your thumb and index finger, and identify the meatus. Using a clean wipe or cotton ball, cleanse first down the middle from the meatus to the rectum, then down each side from the meatus to the rectum, using a clean swab each time.	
b. *For males*—Retract the foreskin, as necessary, and lift the penis perpendicular to the child's body. Cleanse from the meatal opening around the penis in a circular motion. Cleanse three times, using a clean wipe each time.	Microorganisms tend to collect under the foreskin. Lifting the penis straightens the urethra.
10. Place the distal end of the catheter into the specimen container.	Prepares for collection of urine.
11. Slowly insert the catheter. If resistance is met or an obstruction is felt, remove the catheter, and select a smaller-size catheter.[8]	Catheter should not be forced, as injury can occur.
12. Hold the catheter in place until the specimen is obtained.	
13. If an indwelling (Foley) catheter is used, inflate the balloon with sterile saline or sterile water, and tape the catheter securely to the child's inner thigh; if obtaining a specimen only, remove the catheter.	Keeps the catheter in the proper place.
14. Cleanse the perineal area with warm water after the procedure is completed, and apply a diaper or underclothing.	Cleansing the perineal area removes the povidone–iodine and prevents staining of the child's underclothing.
15. Encourage the parent to comfort the child after the procedure; praise the child for cooperating.	
16. Document the time of catheterization; the size of the catheter or feeding tube; the amount, color, and odor of the urine obtained; the type of laboratory analysis performed on the specimen; and how the child tolerated the procedure.	Communicates the nursing interventions and observations to health-care professionals.

REFERENCES

1. Waechter EH, Phillips J, Holaday B. Nursing care of children. 10th ed. Philadelphia: J.B. Lippincott, 1985:83.
2. Hamilton JR. The gastrointestinal tract. In: Behrman RE, Vaughn VC, eds. Nelson textbook of pediatrics. 13th ed. Philadelphia: W.B. Saunders, 1987:767.
3. Bergstern JM, Michael AF. The urinary system. In: Behrman RE, Vaughan VC, eds. Nelson textbook of pediatrics. 13th ed. Philadelphia: W.B. Saunders, 1987:1112.
4. Lutz W. Assessment of the child's health status. In: Servonsky J, Opas SR, eds. Nursing management of children. Boston: Jones & Bartlett, 1987:101.
5. Fleisher GR. Infectious disease emergencies. In: Fleisher G, Ludwig S, eds. Textbook of pediatric emergency medicine. 2nd ed. Baltimore: Williams & Wilkins, 1988;447.
6. Tucker JA, Sussman-Karten K. Treating acute diarrhea and dehydration with an oral solution. Pediatr Nurs 1987;13:172, 174.
7. Sperhac A. Gastrointestinal emergencies. In: Kelly S, ed. Pediatric emergency nursing. Norwalk, CT: Appleton & Lange, 1988:362.
8. Ruddy RM. Illustrated techniques of pediatric emergency procedures. In: Fleisher G, Ludwig S, eds. Textbook of pediatric emergency medicine. 2nd ed. Baltimore: Williams & Wilkins, 1988:1299, 1303, 1307, 1309.
9. Simon R, Brenner BE. Emergency procedures and techniques. 2nd ed. Baltimore: Williams & Wilkins, 1987:13, 345, 347.
10. Henretig FM, Cupit GC, Temple AR, Collins M. Toxicologic emergencies. In: Fleisher G, Ludwig S, eds. Textbook of pediatric emergency medicine. 2nd ed. Baltimore: Williams & Wilkins, 1988:550.
11. Kelly S. Multiple trauma. In: Kelly S, ed. Pediatric emergency nursing. Baltimore: Williams & Wilkins, 1988:133, 138.
12. Committee on Trauma, American College of Surgeons. Advanced Trauma Life Support Student Manual. Chicago: American College of Surgeons, 1989:231.

8

Procedures Involving the Neurological System

Stacey Lang

OVERVIEW OF PEDIATRIC NEUROLOGICAL DIFFERENCES

Two important neurological differences in children are the growing head and brain tissue and the immature spinal column. The infant's head is proportionally larger than the body. The infant's skull is malleable, which makes the brain susceptible to injury. Cerebral tissues are soft, thin and flexible as compared with those of adults.[1] The sulci deepen during childhood, and myleinization continues to occur.

The pediatric spine is immature and elastic, making it easily deformable. Therefore, spinal cord injury in children, unlike adults, frequently occurs without vertebral fracture or dislocation. Momentary intersegmental displacement by external forces endangers the spinal cord without disrupting the bones or ligaments.[2] The resultant spinal cord injury is called SCIWORA (Spinal Cord Injury With Out Radiographic Abnormality).[2] Hyperextension, flexion, distraction and spinal cord ischemia are four potential mechanisms involved with a SCIWORA injury.

Identification of the actual mechanism of injury through thorough history taking is the single best way to identify a SCIWORA injury. Symptoms include complaints of numbness, tingling, weakness, or shooting sensations in the extremities. Oftentimes, the child experiences a transient weakness in the extremities that resolves prior to arrival in the Emergency Department.

Proper diagnosis and treatment of SCIWORA is critical because children who suffer a second injury have a poorer prognosis.[2] Treatment consists of complete cervical immobilization, usually for 3 months.

SPINAL IMMOBILIZATION

Indications Spinal immobilization is indicated in any injured child who has a neurological deficit; who complains of pain in the head, neck or back; who is unconscious or has an altered mental status; who has facial or head injuries; who experienced deceleration forces.[3]

Contraindications   None. However, children presenting to the ED in traumatic arrest, or who require rapid extrication from a private vehicle due to life-threatening conditions, must be quickly immobilized, using whatever means possible.

Complications   Further spinal cord injury if spinal immobilization is not adequately maintained or is improperly applied.

Equipment

> Commercially available pediatric immobilization device
> Commercially available cervical immobilization device (CID)
> Prepared half back board
> Papoose board
> Exam table or a flat surface
> Towel or blanket rolls
> 1″ adhesive tape
> Rigid cervical collars—all sizes
> Prepared long back board
> Gloves

Psychosocial Considerations   The injured child with spinal immobilization may have fears and guilt for participating in a forbidden activity that led to the trauma. The simultaneous performance of other procedures (blood pressure [BP] measurement, intravenous [IV] insertion, and so forth) heightens the child's anxiety. Keep in the child's line of vision, touch the child while speaking to him or her, and maintain eye contact; these actions allow the child to focus on the emergency nurse for support. Standing directly over the child's face is threatening and should be avoided. Release the child from the immobilization devices as soon as a spinal injury has been ruled out.

Parents should receive simple explanations regarding the reasons for and methods of immobilization. If at all possible, parents should be allowed to provide comfort and distraction if they are emotionally capable of doing so.

Nursing responsibilities are described in Table 8.1.

Table 8.1.   Nursing Responsibilities

NURSING ACTIONS	RATIONALE
1. Explain to the child and the family the need for spinal immobilization. Instruct the child to remain still.	Enhances their understanding and cooperation.
2. Don gloves; stand or kneel behind the child's head. Place one hand on each side of the child's head, with the thumbs placed directly behind the ears and the forefingers extending along the angle of the jaw. Use the jaw thrust if necessary to maintain a patent airway. (See Chapter 4.)	Provides manual immobilization; ensures the child's safety prior to placement of the immobilization device.

Table 8.1. (*cont.*)

NURSING ACTIONS	RATIONALE
3. Either transfer manual stabilization to another health professional or instruct the other health professional to perform the primary and secondary trauma surveys. Do *not* apply manual traction unless instructed to do so by the physician.	Provides baseline information on the child's condition. Manual traction could cause a distraction injury to the spinal cord in the child with an unstable cervical spine.
4. While standing or kneeling at the child's head, continuously assess the head and neck position; talk calmly to the child and remind her or him to remain still.	Assures that the head is in a neutral midline position.
5. Have another health professional apply a rigid collar while manually stabilizing the neck in a neutral position.	An inappropriate size of collar does not provide adequate cervical immobilization. A proper size of collar supports the mandible and occipit.
a. *If the child is sitting,* slide the one piece collar up the chest wall so that the child's chin is supported by the chin piece. Bring the back portion behind the neck and secure with the Velcro® straps.	
b. *If the child is supine,* slide the back portion of the collar behind and around the child's neck. Bring the chin piece to the child's chin, and secure with the Velcro® straps.	
In either case, the sides of the collar should not cover the ears.	
6. Place the prepared backboard parallel to the child; remove the foam CID blocks.	A prepared long backboard has an attached CID and 3 9-foot straps.
7. Instruct the child to keep her or his arms at the sides.	
8. Place the child on the backboard while maintaining manual immobilization. While positioning the child on the backboard, examine the scalp, neck, and back and buttocks, and remove debris that could cause further trauma to the skin (e.g., cinders, glass, dirt).	Prevents trauma to the skin that could occur through prolonged immobilization.
a. *For the child in a supine position,* log roll the child, as a unit, onto his or her side. Slide the backboard under the child and tilt it	

Table 8.1.   (*cont.*)

NURSING ACTIONS	RATIONALE
against the child's back at a 30–45° angle.[3] Roll the child back onto the board.[3] Ensure that the cervical spine is kept midline; ensure midline placement by drawing an imaginary line from the child's nose to the sternum. While log rolling, keep the child's nose in line with the sternum. Secure the child with the attached straps (see Step 9).	
b. *For the child in an upright position* (such as being held against a parent, or standing upright), bring the prepared backboard up to the child's back snugly. Lower the board and the child to a supine position. Secure the child with the straps (see Step 9).	
c. *For the child in a sitting position* (such as in a chair or a private vehicle), slip a prepared half backboard behind the child. Bring the lower straps over each leg, down between both legs, and back around the outside of the same leg.[3] Bring the straps upward across the chest and attach them to the opposite upper straps that were brought over the shoulders.[3] Tighten the straps until the child is secure.[3]	A prepared half backboard has crisscrossed straps behind the board with the top straps across the shoulders and the bottom straps exiting through the lower-most side holes.
Secure the child's head to the board with wide tape; use padding to fill the void behind the neck.[3]	Maintains a neutral position.[3]
Slide the end of the long backboard under the child's buttocks. Place the child so the half backboard lies flat upon the long backboard. Slide the child up into position on the long backboard, supporting the legs at a 90° angle to the torso. Loosen the straps to extend the legs flat, then retighten them.[3] Secure the child to the long backboard using the long board straps and a CID.[3]	The half backboard is a splint and is not used as a handle to move the child.[3]
9. Secure the child to the long backboard.	

Table 8.1.   (*cont.*)

NURSING ACTIONS	RATIONALE
a. Loop the first 9-foot strap underneath the handhold nearest the child's shoulder. Route the strap diagonally toward the contralateral hip and loop it through a handhold near this hip. Bring the end of this strap back across the child's torso, and connect it to the other end of this strap.	
b. The second 9-foot strap is applied using the same technique beginning at the opposite shoulder, resulting in a crisscross pattern.	
c. The third 9-foot strap is looped underneath the handhold near the child's knees. This strap is laid across the lower extremities, looped through the opposite handhold, and laid back upon itself and connected.	
d. An alternative method is to apply the straps as demonstrated in Figure 8.1.	

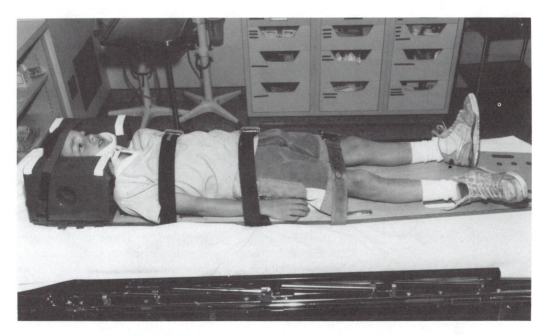

Figure 8.1. Spinal immobilization on a long backboard. Straps are fastened snugly around the child's torso to maintain proper spinal alignment. If the patient vomits, the child and long backboard are tilted laterally as a unit.

Table 8.1.   *(cont.)*

NURSING ACTIONS	RATIONALE

e. Immobilizing an infant in a car seat is demonstrated in Figure 8.2.

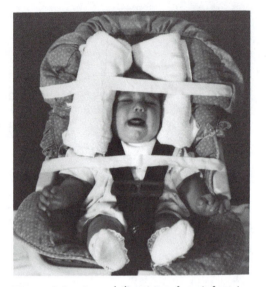

Figure 8.2.   Immobilization of an infant in a car seat. The infant should remain strapped in the car seat until spinal injury is ruled out. Place one large towel in a horseshoe shape over the child's head to the shoulders. Or, as illustrated, place two small towels on either side of the neck and over the head. Secure the towel(s) with one inch tape starting at one side of the car seat, crossing the infant's forehead. Anchor the tape at the other side of the car seat. Place additional one-inch tape in the same fashion across the infant's chest. Use additional small towels to fill in any voids in the car seat.

f. When immobilizing a child in a commercially available pediatric immobilization device, follow the manufacturer's instructions.

g. Apply the foam cushions of the CID and place the head strap across the child's forehead. The chin strap is not used in children (see Figure 8.3).

The chin strap can push the jaw backward, potentially obstructing the airway or may further compromise the child's airway and increase the risk of aspiration, should emesis occur.

Table 8.1.   *(cont.)*

NURSING ACTIONS	RATIONALE

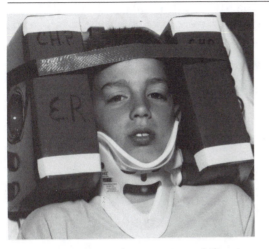

Figure 8.3. Cervical spine immobilization with cervical immobilization device (CID). Note that the chin strap is not used, due to potential risk of airway compromise.

NURSING ACTIONS	RATIONALE
10. If using towels, place one on each side of the child's head so that they are resting against the side of the face and head. Using adhesive tape, secure the towels to the head by taping from the backboard and across the child's forehead to the other side of the backboard.	Provides immobilization to the cervical spine.
11. Assess the child's tolerance to the immobilization, and reassess the child's neurological functioning.	Detects possible complications of immobilization.
12. Document the time of immobilization, the size of the rigid collar, the findings of the primary and secondary surveys, and any changes in the pre- and postimmobilization neurological assessments.	Communicates nursing interventions and observations to health-care professionals.

ASSISTING WITH APPLICATION OF GARDNER–WELLS TONGS

Indications   Gardner–Wells Tongs are indicated to stabilize and realign an unstable cervical spine when immediate fusion or placement of a halo apparatus is inappropriate, due to muscle spasm or poor skeletal alignment.

Contraindications   Children less than 6 years of age are not candidates for the tongs because the skull table is too thin.[4] Gardner–Wells tongs should not be used when the cervical spine is extremely unstable, e.g., when free bone chips are evident on the cervical spine x-ray.

Complications   So-called ping-pong fracture (minimally depressed skull fracture) in an infant;[4] a depressed skull fracture in children less than 6 years of age;[4] infection;[4] intracranial hematoma.[4]

Equipment

> 1% lidocaine for injection local anesthetic
> One 3-cc syringe with a 25-gauge needle
> Disposable razor
> Povidone–iodine solution
> Gardner–Wells tongs
> Skeletal traction rope (4–5 ft)
> Weights
> Stryker Frame or Rotorest™ Bed
> Povidone–iodine scrub
> Gloves
> Antispasmodic or sedation agents

Psychosocial Considerations   Placement of skeletal traction can be frightening for the child and family, due to the procedure and the appearance of the tongs. The child and parents may have difficulty understanding anatomically where the tongs are placed and may think that the tongs enter the brain. Tong placement requires the child to remain supine for a prolonged period of time which may precipitate anxiety in the child and the family. Thorough but simple explanations of the location of the tongs and the reasons for placement help to alleviate their fears. A model of the skull is helpful in explaining the location of the tongs. Deep breathing exercises during placement of the tongs may help to calm the child and to achieve some degree of cooperation, as will the judicious use of sedation agents.

Parents may be present for the procedure if the staff feel comfortable inserting the tongs in the parents' presence and if the parents' presence is likely to comfort the child.

Nursing responsibilities are described in Table 8.2.

Table 8.2. Nursing Responsibilities

NURSING ACTIONS	RATIONALE
1. Explain to the child and family the need for the Gardner–Wells tongs.	Enhances their understanding and cooperation.
2. Perform a complete neurological assessment. Administer antispasmodic or sedation agents, as ordered by the physician. Assess sedative effects on airway and respiratory status. Don gloves.	Provides a baseline of the child's condition.
3. The physician identifies the insertion sites. Landmarks for identification of the insertion site are above the pinnae of the ears on an imagi-	Allows traction to place the cervical spine in a neutral position.

Table 8.2. (*cont.*)

NURSING ACTIONS	RATIONALE
nary plane connecting the mastoid processes with the external auditory canal.[5]	
4. Prepare the insertion site by scrubbing the area with povidone–iodine scrub and shaving 2 cm × 2 cm area of the scalp.	Decreases risk of infection.
5. The physician injects 1% lidocaine at the sites where the tongs are inserted.	Decreases pain.
6. Apply manual traction or assist with manual traction, as directed by the physician while tongs are inserted. Manual traction is applied while standing at the head of the child's bed and supporting the head at the angle of the jaw bilaterally. Forefingers are placed along the jaw line with the thumbs extending behind the ear.	Provides stability for the upper cervical cord.
Great care should be taken not to allow either flexion or extension of the neck.	Reduces risk of additional spinal-cord injury.
7. The physician inserts the tongs, with a gentle, slow, twisting motion. Placement is checked every 3–5 mm, and advancement halts when the pins are firmly seated in the bone. The button safety device should be observed for any indication of penetration through the inner table of the skull. This penetration has occurred if the button is no longer flush with the tongs.	Minimizes risk of associated complications.
8. After the tongs are inserted, the physician applies manual traction by holding the tongs. At this time, the child is moved with extreme care onto the Stryker Frame or Rotorest™ Bed.	Necessitates only one move for the child with an unstable cervical spine.
9. Attach the rope and weights to the tongs, as directed by the physician. Weights are calculated by counting from the occiput to the upper unstable segment at 2 lb of weight per segment.[4] Increments of 2 lb each are added, as desired, up to a maximum equivalent to 25% of the child's body weight.[4] Weights are re-	Avoids sudden jarring motions that could cause further trauma to the spine.

Table 8.2.   (*cont.*)

NURSING ACTIONS	RATIONALE
leased very slowly once they are attached to the child.	
10. Observe for muscle spasm or voluntary contraction of the muscles of the neck and shoulders. Repeat the neurological assessment.	May render cervical traction ineffective and require the use of additional weights and/or muscle relaxants.
11. Obtain a lateral cervical spine x-ray film after each manipulation of the weights and traction axis.[4]	Determines the effectiveness of the traction.
12. Document the time of tong application, the child's tolerance for and response to the placement of the tongs, the neurological assessment before and after tong placement, the amount of weights applied, the x-ray findings, the type of bed onto which the child was moved, and whether any muscle relaxants/sedatives were administered.	Communicates the nursing interventions and observations to health-care professionals.

ASSISTING WITH LUMBAR PUNCTURE

Indications   Lumbar puncture (LP) is performed as a diagnostic test in children with suspected meningitis, meningoencephalitis, subarachnoid hemorrhage or other neurological syndromes.[6] In addition, this procedure is occasionally used for the administration of medications. The lumbar puncture involves the passing of a needle into the subarachnoid space to obtain cerebrospinal fluid (CSF) for diagnostic study.

Contraindications   Signs of increased intracranial pressure (ICP). A history of poorly treated hydrocephalus or physical findings of increased ICP may necessitate the performance of a computed tomography (CT) scan prior to the lumbar puncture.

Complications   Brainstem herniation; pain at the insertion site; headache; bleeding from the insertion site; CSF leakage.

Equipment

> LP tray
> > 2 sterile drapes (1 plain, 1 fenestrated)
> > Sterile gauze sponges
> > Forceps
> > 4 specimen tubes
> > Pressure manometer
> 2 cups for antiseptic solutions (povidone–iodine solution; isopropyl alcohol)
> Spinal needle
> > 22-gauge 1–1½" for children < 1 year (may use for small or thin toddler)
> > 22-gauge 2½" for children > 1 year

Sterile gloves
1% lidocaine for local anesthetic
Sterile 3-cc syringe with a 25-gauge needle for anesthetic infiltration
Band-Aid™
Mask (if bacterial meningitis is suspected)

Psychosocial Considerations   Explain the procedure to the child, using developmentally appropriate language. Explain to the child that he or she will be held snugly and that his or her job is to hold very still. Sometimes pain occurs in the legs from stimulation of the nerve roots and may be relieved by repositioning the child or the needle. Encourage the child to tell you if he or she has any discomfort or pain. Honestly answer any questions the child may have. These reassuring measures may help to lessen the child's anxiety during the procedure. Parents may be present for the LP if the staff feels comfortable performing the procedure in the parents' presence, and if the parents' presence is likely to comfort the child.

Nursing responsibilities are described in Table 8.3.

Table 8.3. Nursing Responsibilities

NURSING ACTIONS	RATIONALE
1. Explain to the child and the family the need for the lumbar puncture. Obtain written consent, in accordance with institutional policy. Assess for previous spinal cord pathology (e.g., myelomeningocele, cord tumor, tethered cord).	Enhances their understanding and cooperation; prevents complications.
2. Position the infant or child for the LP.	
a. Place the child in the lateral decubitus position, with the child's knees drawn up to the abdomen and the neck flexed forward. Secure the child in this position throughout the procedure, ensuring that the child's shoulders and hips are perpendicular to the stretcher/exam table. Place one arm over the child's neck and the other behind the child's knees[7] (see Figure 8.4).	This position widens the lumbar space and provides easy access for the spinal needle.
b. Alternatively, the upright position may be used in infants. The infant is placed in a sitting position with his or her thighs against the abdomen and the neck flexed forward.[7] The holder stabilizes the infant against his or her upper torso and immobilizes the infant's extremities[7] (see Fig-	

Table 8.3.   (*cont.*)

NURSING ACTIONS	RATIONALE

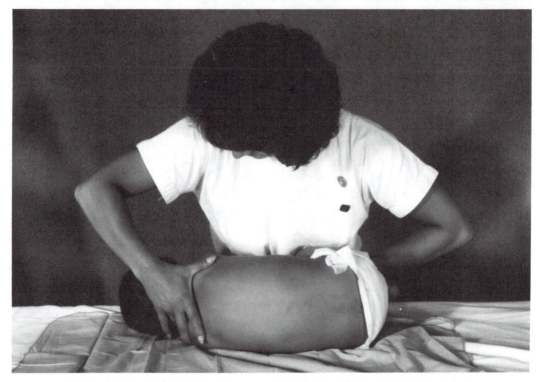

Figure 8.4.   Positioning the young child in the left lateral decubitus position for a lumbar puncture (LP). Note how the nurse is able to observe the child's reactions, as well as to provide emotional support verbally. An alternative method is to place your left arm beneath the child's thighs and to grasp his or her wrists—this restrains both the arms and the legs.

NURSING ACTIONS	RATIONALE
ure 8.5 (a) and (b)). This upright position may also be used in the child with difficult access (e.g., narrowed lumbar spaces or obesity) or in children displaying symptoms of respiratory distress. In such cases, the child is positioned with the legs dangling over the edge of the stretcher, with the torso slightly bent forward at the waist.	
Avoid hyperflexion of the neck in children less than 1 year of age; caution must be exercised to avoid vigorous holding.	Hyperflexion can increase the risk of respiratory compromise. Vigorous holding may lead to cardiopulmonary arrest.[7]
3. The physician locates the site for the LP by identifying the spinous process immediately below or lateral to	Locates proper site for needle insertion.

Table 8.3. *(cont.)*

NURSING ACTIONS	RATIONALE

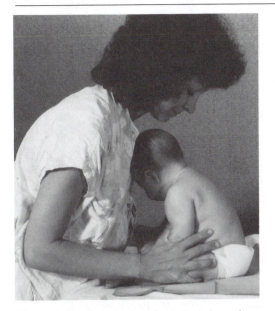

Figure 8.5. Positioning the infant for a lumbar puncture. This is an alternative to the lateral decubitus position. The infant's arms and legs are secured by the nurse's hands, while the infant's head rests on the nurse's chest. Ideally, the infant's head should be midline: (a) side view; (b) back view.

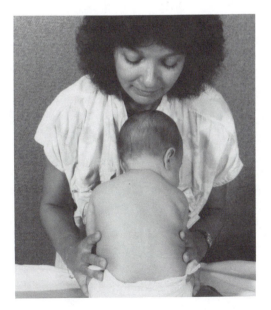

Table 8.3.   (*cont.*)

NURSING ACTIONS	RATIONALE
the iliac crest (interspaces L3–L4 or L4–L5). These landmarks may not be helpful in the child with spinal cord pathology, and an alternative puncture site may be chosen.	
4. The physician cleanses the child's back with povidone–iodine and alcohol. If a diaper is present, fold it down enough to expose the sacral area while keeping the rectal area covered.	Prevents contamination of the sterile field from feces.
5. The physician places the plain sterile drape under the child and the fenestrated drape across the child's back, with the opening over the lumbar area.	Creates a sterile field.
6. The physician injects 1% lidocaine in children older than 1 year of age.[6]	Decreases pain during needle insertion.
7. The physician inserts the needle bevel up into the subarachnoid space, aiming toward the umbilicus. The stylet is removed. Attach the manometer, if desired.	Allows for the collection of a specimen. Manometer measures the fluid pressure.
8. The physician collects approximately 1 cc of CSF for analysis in each of four numbered specimen tubes. Send the CSF specimens to the lab for the following studies: Tube #1 Culture and sensitivity and Gram stain (STAT) Tube #2 Protein and glucose (STAT) Tube #3 Cell count (STAT) Tube #4 Hold for further studies if indicated (viral studies may require special media)	
9. The physician reinserts the stylet and removes the needle.	
10. The physician applies pressure to the puncture site with a sterile 2 × 2 gauze pad, and applies a Band-Aid™.	
11. Praise the child for cooperating.	Provides reassurance and sense of mastery.
12. Remove any cleansing agent from the child's back.	Promotes comfort.
13. Instruct the older child/adolescent to lie flat.	Minimizes the risk of post-LP headache.

Table 8.3. (*cont.*)

NURSING ACTIONS	RATIONALE
The younger child and infant may be held by the parent in a position of comfort.	Headaches following LP are more common in adults.[7]
14. Document the child's and the parent's understanding of the procedure, the size of the needle, the administration of a local anesthetic, the site of needle insertion, the character of the CSF, the child's tolerance of the procedure, any complications, and the laboratory analyses and results.	Communicates the nursing interventions and observations to health-care professionals.

ASSISTING WITH VENTRICULAR TAP

Indications A ventricular tap is performed to remove CSF from the ventricles in emergent situations (e.g., central herniation) when rapid decompression of the brain stem is vital, or for diagnostic purposes (e.g., suspected ventriculitis). A ventricular tap is most commonly performed on infants, as this procedure requires that the anterior fontanel be open. In rare cases, a ventricular tap may be accomplished in an older child (less than 3 years of age), when the situation does not allow time for a formal ventriculostomy. In the Emergency Department, this procedure is reserved for extremely urgent situations in which the CSF must be removed quickly, to alleviate increased intracranial pressure.

Contraindications Not usually performed in children with a closed anterior fontanel. In addition, children with congenital abnormalities of the central nervous system (CNS) may not be acceptable candidates, as the ventricular size and location may make access during a ventricular tap impossible.

Complications Trauma to the brain tissues and blood vessels; entrance of the needle into the superior sagittal sinus;[8] bleeding; infection.

Equipment

> Povidone–iodine solution
> Povidone–iodine scrub
> Lidocaine
> Sterile gloves
> Sterile drapes
> Sterile 4 × 4 gauze sponges
> One 22-gauge 2½″ spinal needle
> Three sterile test tubes
> Pressure manometer, if desired
> Three-way stopclock

The foregoing items may be available in a prepackaged, disposable LP tray. In addition, obtain the following:

Disposable razor
Adhesive tape
Sheet for use as a restraint (if necessary)
Povidone–iodine ointment

Psychosocial Considerations A warm room and a soft, calming voice promote the infant's comfort. Application of a mummy-type restraint system may also assist in securing the child. The parents should be provided with concise and accurate information about what the procedure entails. Parents should also be reassured that insertion of the needle itself does not cause damage to the brain tissue.

Nursing responsibilities are described in Table 8.4.

Table 8.4.   Nursing Responsibilities

NURSING ACTIONS	RATIONALE
1. Explain the procedure to the family. Time may not permit for this preparation.	Enhances the family's understanding.
2. Perform a neurological assessment.	Provides a baseline of the child's condition.
3. Don gloves and restrain the child. It is desirable to have one person solely responsible for restraint.	Prevents contamination of field and decreases the risk of movement once the needle has been inserted.
Restraint is best accomplished by the application of a mummy-type restraint. The head is held between the palms of the two hands, with the fingers interlocked behind the occiput.	Minimizes lateral movement of the head during the procedure.
4. The physician selects the puncture site. Ventricular tap is usually accomplished through the frontal horn of the right lateral ventricle. This is most easily located at the coronal suture, midpupillary line, in line with the tragus.	The right brain is preferred because the majority of people are left-brain dominant.
5. Prepare the site by cleansing with povidone–iodine scrub and shaving the hair. A 6 × 6 cm area should be shaved. Great care is taken to avoid nicking the skin during shaving.	Minimizes the risk of infection.
Remove stray hair from the site after shaving by patting the area with a strip of adhesive tape.	Reduces the risk of contamination of the field.
6. The physician inserts the needle slowly, in line with the previously described landmarks. The needle is advanced by only 1–2 mm at a time,	Minimizes risk of trauma to the brain tissue due to overinsertion of the needle.

Table 8.4.   (*cont.*)

NURSING ACTIONS	RATIONALE
after which the stylet is removed and the free flow of CSF is ascertained. The fluid pressure should be measured, if ordered by the physician.	
7. After the tap, apply a pressure dressing to the site, and elevate the head of the bed. Use povidone–iodine ointment, a 4 × 4 gauze pad, folded into fourths, and adhesive tape. Repeat the neurological assessment.	Helps to prevent CSF leak.
8. Send the CSF for tests, as ordered by the physician.	Aids in diagnosis of the disease process.
9. Document the site of the tap, as well as the appearance of the fluid, the amount removed, the pressure reading, the specimens sent, the neurological assessments before and after the tap, and the infant's tolerance of the procedure.	Communicates the nursing interventions and observations to health-care professionals.

HELMET REMOVAL

Indications   Helmets are removed if the airway or neutral alignment of the cervical spine cannot be maintained.

Contraindications   Helmets should not be removed if the child complains of pain during removal attempts.[9] If the patient is unconscious, it may be difficult to remove the helmet.[9]

Complications   Aggravation of a head or cervical spine injury.[9]

Equipment

>Prepared long backboard
>CID
>Rigid cervical collars—all sizes
>Gloves

Psychosocial Considerations   For children and adolescents who suffer a sports-related injury, their primary concern may be their future ability to participate in sports. The adolescent, injured on a motorcycle or all-terrain vehicle (ATV), may have concerns about future operation of these vehicles. Gaining the child's cooperation may be difficult with a concomitant head injury. Reassuring the child and family and explaining the treatment process enhances their coping abilities.

>Nursing responsibilities are described in Table 8.5.

Table 8.5. Nursing Responsibilities

NURSING ACTIONS	RATIONALE
1. Explain to the child and the family the need for helmet removal.	Enhances their understanding and cooperation.
2. Perform a neurological assessment.	Provides a baseline of the child's condition.
3. Don gloves. Position the first health professional at the child's head. The first health professional applies in-line cervical stabilization by placing his or her hands on each side of the helmet, with the fingers on the child's neck and on the mandible.[3] Position the second health professional at the child's shoulders.	Prevents slippage of the helmet.[9]
4. The second health professional removes the chin strap while the first health professional maintains in-line stabilization.[3]	
5. The second health professional assumes responsibility for cervical immobilization. He or she places one hand behind the child's neck on the occipital ridge while the thumb and index finger of the other hand supports the mandible.[3]	
6. The first health professional removes the helmet by expanding it laterally and pulling it gently over the child's ears.[3] Remove the child's eyeglasses if the helmet is a full-face helmet.[3] With a full-face helmet, tilt it backward during removal, to avoid injuring the nose. The second health professional maintains cervical stabilization as the helmet is removed.	Prevents head tilt.[3]
7. After the helmet is removed, the first health professional resumes responsibility for cervical immobilization. He or she places one hand on each side of the child's head, with the thumbs placed directly behind the ears and the forefingers extending along the angle of the jaw. Assess the head and neck for soft tissue injuries, foreign bodies, and so forth.	Maintains in-line cervical stabilization.
8. Initiate cervical and spinal immobilization procedures. (Refer to Table 8.1).	

Table 8.5.   *(cont.)*

NURSING ACTIONS	RATIONALE
9. Repeat the neurological assessment.	Determines whether any neurological changes have occurred during the procedure.
10. Document the type of helmet, the time of removal, the neurological assessments before and after the removal, and how the child tolerated the procedure.	Communicates the nursing interventions and observations to health-care professionals.

REFERENCES

1. Thompson S. Emergency care of children. Boston: Jones and Bartlett, 1990:166.
2. Pang D, Pollack I. Spinal cord injury without radiographic abnormality in children: The SCIWORA syndrome. J Trauma 1989;29:654, 660.
3. Campbell JE. ed. Basic trauma life support: Advanced prehospital care. 2nd ed. Englewood Cliffs, NJ: Prentice Hall, 1988:271–272, 275–276, 288, 311–313.
4. Pang D, Hanley EN. Special problems of spinal stabilization in children. In: Cooper PR, ed. Management of posttraumatic spinal instability. Park Ridge, IL: American Association of Neurological Surgeons, 1990:184–186.
5. Chestnut RM, Marshall LF. Early assessment, transport, and management of patients with posttraumatic spinal instability. In: Cooper PR, ed. Management of posttraumatic spinal instability. Park Ridge, IL: American Association of Neurological Surgeons, 1990:9.
6. Ruddy RM (section ed). Procedures: Illustrated techniques of pediatric emergency procedures. In: Fleisher GR, Ludwig S, eds. Textbook of pediatric emergency medicine. 2nd ed. Baltimore: Williams & Wilkins, 1988:1270.
7. King E, Wieck L, Dyer M. Quick reference to pediatric nursing procedures. Philadelphia: JB Lippincott, 1983:143.
8. Hughes W, Buescher E. Pediatric procedures. 2nd ed. Philadelphia: W.B. Saunders, 1980:186.
9. Hafen BQ, Karren KJ. Prehospital, emergency care and crisis intervention. 2nd ed. Englewood, CO: Morton Publishing, 1983:276–277.

9

Procedures Involving the Musculoskeletal System

Rita Dello-Stritto

OVERVIEW OF PEDIATRIC MUSCULOSKELETAL DIFFERENCES

The musculoskeletal system consists of bone, muscles, ligaments, tendons, and joints. Together these tissues provide for movement, support, and structure of the body and protection of the vital organs.[1] *Tendons* attach muscles to bones, whereas the *ligaments* connect bone to bone; when working together properly, they produce movement at the joints.

The basic difference between the skeleton of the child and that of the adult is the presence of the epiphyseal plate (growth cartilage or growth plate), which is responsible for longitudinal bone growth in the child. It is a radiolucent cartilaginous disc found between the epiphysis and metaphysis, located at both the distal and proximal ends of long bones.[2] Injury to the epiphyseal plate may result in growth cessation; therefore, the younger the child is at the time of an injury, the shorter the limb will be in adult life.[3]

The bones of the child are characteristically more flexible than those of the adult; in addition, the child's periosteum is much thicker and stronger. As a result, some fractures in children are incomplete and leave the periosteum intact on one side. This condition is referred to as a "greenstick fracture."[2]

The periosteal covering of the child's bone is capable of rapid production of callus (new bone) over a short period of time. This covering allows fractures to heal rapidly but also affords the clinician a shorter period of time to perform definitive reduction of the fracture.

SLING AND SWATH

Indications   The sling and swath are used to help stabilize fractures or dislocations of an upper extremity. They are also useful in stabilizing injuries to the clavicle and for anterior dislocations of the shoulder.[4] The sling and swath are fashioned from two triangular bandages or are purchased as a complete unit (often called an "arm immobilizer").

Contraindications   None.

Complications   Impaired circulation if the sling and swath are not properly applied.

Equipment

> 2 triangular bandages
> 2 × 2 gauze pads
> Safety pins or tape
> Commercially available arm immobilizer

Psychosocial Considerations   The sling and swath limits mobility in the child at a time when mobility is used to communicate to others and master development tasks. The child may experience frustration by physical limitations. For some children, loss of mobility can have a negative impact on their sense of self-esteem. These considerations can be conveyed to the family so that they can understand how to be prepared for some possible acting-out or regressive behaviors at home.

Nursing responsibilities are described in Table 9.1.

Table 9.1.   Nursing Responsibilities

NURSING ACTIONS	RATIONALE
1. Explain to the child and the family the need for the sling and swath.	Enhances their understanding and cooperation.
2. Assess the child's neurovascular status: distal pulses, capillary refill, color, and sensation. Do not straighten any angulation of a bone or joint in order to place a sling and swath, unless circulation and/or nerve function are impaired.[4]	Provides a baseline neurovascular assessment; realignment can cause further damage to the injured arm.
3. Position the largest angle of the triangular bandage behind the elbow.[5]	
4. Bring the bottom point of the triangle up and over the arm and shoulder of the injured arm.[5]	
5. Bring the two ends together and tie. Ensure that the child's hand is elevated 4 inches above the elbow.[5]	Allows for elevation of the arm to minimize pain and swelling.
6. Check the child's distal pulse, color, capillary refill, and sensation.	Ensures that placement of the sling did not impair circulation or nerve function.
7. Take the point of the bandage at the elbow, and fold it forward, pinning or taping it to the front of the sling. If no pin is available, tie a knot in the point[5] (see Figure 9.1).	This action forms a pocket in which the elbow can rest and ensures that the elbow will not slip out of the sling.

Table 9.1.   (*cont.*)

NURSING ACTIONS	RATIONALE

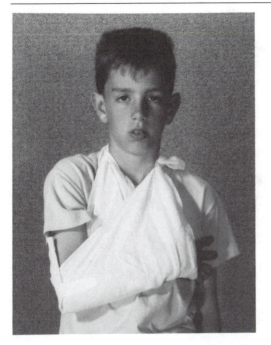

Figure 9.1. Placement of an arm sling: The arm is positioned at the heart level. The elbow corner is secured with tape instead of a pin, and the knot is on the shoulder to prevent irritation to the neck.

8. Fold the second triangular bandage lengthwise several times to form a long swath.

9. Tie the swath around the chest and the injured arm over the sling. *Do not* place the swath over the uninjured arm[5] (see Figure 9.2).

Stabilizes the upper extremity against the chest wall.

Table 9.1. *(cont.)*

NURSING ACTIONS	RATIONALE

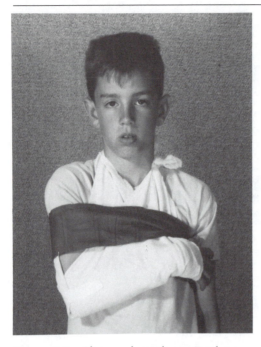

Figure 9.2. Sling and swath are in place.

NURSING ACTIONS	RATIONALE
10. Reassess the child's neurovascular status.	Ensures that the repositioning of the arm did not impair distal circulation or nerve function.
11. Place padding under each knot that comes in contact with the child's skin.	Helps to prevent skin breakdown.
12. Document the child's neurovascular status before and after sling-and-swath placement, as well as the time of placement. Teach the family how to position the sling and swath at home.	Communicates the nursing interventions and observations to health-care professionals.

SPLINTING

Indications   Splinting is indicated to immobilize a suspected fracture of an extremity. It is used primarily as an initial, rather than definitive, treatment. A splint prevents a closed fracture from becoming an open fracture and minimizes damage to nerves, blood vessels, muscles, and bone ends. Splinting also reduces pain, prevents soft tissue damage, and allows for safe transportation of the child.[5] Splints are also used to immobilize the injured extremity until initial swelling has been reduced and casting has been applied. This reduction of swelling often takes 3–5 days.

Type of Splints and Use

1. *Rigid splint*—A nonflexible device secured to a fractured extremity to help maintain stability. Splints are made of heavy cardboard, padded board, aluminum, plaster, wood, and so on. The splint should be wide enough and long enough to extend distally and proximally to the suspected fracture site.[4]
2. *Air splint*—A device that uses air pressure to maintain stabilization of a fracture site. The splint is inflated by mouth in the same way that a balloon is inflated. Air splints are best suited for suspected fractures of the lower leg and of the forearm.[4]
3. *Traction splint*—The traction splint is used only to maintain a constant pull on the lower extremity when a femur or hip fracture is suspected. The traction helps to keep the ends of the bones from overlapping, due to muscle contraction. The traction splint is *not* used to reduce the fracture.[4]
4. *Vacuum splint*—A styrofoam bead-filled device that, when its air is evacuated, creates a form-fitting splint.

Contraindications   Splints are not used if their placement impairs the distal circulation of the injured extremity.

Complications   Impaired neurovascular status.

Equipment

> Correct size and type of splint
> Padding
> Tape
> Roller gauze
> Gloves

Psychosocial Considerations   The splint provides temporary relief from the pain and discomfort associated with the injury. Young children may be frightened by the splint application procedure or by thinking that the arm or leg is gone. Simple explanations of how the splint is applied, how the splint works, and why it is needed should help to allay the child's anxiety.

Parents, too, need to understand that the splint is to help the child until definitive care is available; they should be encouraged to comfort their child while waiting for treatment.

Nursing responsibilities are described in Table 9.2.

Table 9.2. Nursing Responsibilities

NURSING ACTIONS	RATIONALE
1. Explain to the child and family the need for the splint. Describe any sensations the child will feel.	Enhances their understanding and cooperation.
2. Cut away or remove any clothing that covers the suspected fracture site.[4]	Allows proper visualization of the suspected fracture site.
3. Assess the child's neurovascular status.	Provides a baseline neurovascular assessment.
4. Cover all wounds with sterile dressings.	Keeps the wound site clean, reduces the chance of infection, and controls bleeding.

Table 9.2.   (*cont.*)

NURSING ACTIONS	RATIONALE
5. If the child has an open fracture, do *not* attempt to replace the exposed bone ends into skin.[4]	Reduces the possibility of further damage and introduction of foreign material into the wound site.
6. *Do not* attempt to straighten fractures involving any joint. Splint the fractures in the position in which they are found.[4]	Straightening a fracture near the joint may cause further damage and may decrease circulation distal to the fracture site.
7. Place a padded splint that extends distally and proximally to the fracture site to immobilize the joint above and below the suspected fracture site.[4]	The padded splint helps to reduce tissue breakdown. Immobilizing the joint above and below the fracture site reduces the chance of converting a closed fracture into an open fracture.
8. If the fracture involves the wrist or forearm, place the hand in a position of function and fill in all spaces between the splint and the extremity with gauze.	Helps reduce the movement of the fracture site.
9. If the fracture is of the lower leg, place a padded splint on either side of, or behind, the leg.	Helps reduce the movement of the fracture site.
10. Using tape, roller gauze, or cloth ties, secure the extremity to the splint. Do *not* cover the fracture site during this process (see Figure 9.3).	Allows for visualization of the fracture site.

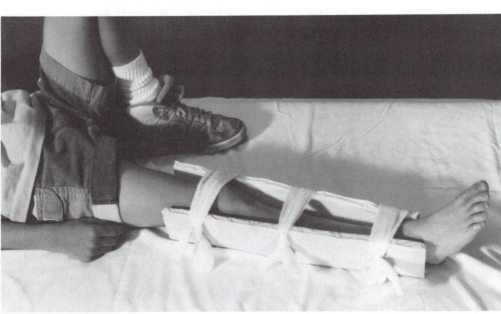

Figure 9.3.   Splint placement for an injured leg. The knots are placed outside the splint to prevent direct pressure on the extremity. Uniform pressure should be applied.

Table 9.2. *(cont.)*

NURSING ACTIONS	RATIONALE
Follow manufacturer's instructions for the application and removal of commercially available splints.	
11. Assess the child's neurovascular status.	Ensures that splint placement did not produce neurovascular compromise.
12. Document the neurovascular status before and after splint application, as well as the time of splint application. Document how the child tolerated the procedure.	Communicates the nursing interventions and observations to health-care professionals.

CRUTCH WALKING

Indications   Crutches are used as adjunctive therapy to mobilize the child when the lower extremity is injured.

Contraindications   Crutch walking should not be used in children who have impaired muscle strength and/or problems with coordination of the upper body.

Complications   Brachial plexus irritation from improperly adjusted crutches; potential injury from incorrect use.

Equipment

> Correct size of crutches
> Rubber crutch tips
> Rubber hand supports
> Rubber axillary pads

Psychosocial Considerations   Once they have practiced with the crutches, children become adept with this new means of mobility. The older child may need reinforcement to use the crutches, as she or he may not wish to seem different from his or her peers; on the other hand, older children and adolescents may use the crutches to gain sympathy from family and friends.

Children of all ages must be taught that crutches are not toys or weapons and must be used only for ambulation. Parents and children should be made aware of the potential harm that could occur if the crutches are not used properly.

Nursing responsibilities are described in Table 9.3.

ASSISTING WITH CAST APPLICATION

Indications   Casting is indicated to immobilize the joints above and below the fracture site. Casting is used to keep fractures and dislocations reduced to support soft-tissue injuries, or to prevent movement in an inflamed or protected area.[7] This technique is recommended when immobilization of an injured extremity is essential to the total healing process.

Table 9.3. Nursing Responsibilities

NURSING ACTIONS	RATIONALE
1. Explain to the child and the family the need for the crutches. Emphasize the importance of their proper use.	Enhances their understanding and cooperation.
2. Ensure that the crutches have rubber tips.[6]	Rubber tips help prevent the crutches from slipping.
3. Adjust the crutch size to the child. The top of the crutches should be approximately 2 finger-widths (2.5 to 3.8 cm) below the axillae.[6]	If the crutches are too high in the axillary region, irritation to the brachial plexus area may occur leading to numbness and tingling of the torso and upper extremities.
4. Adjust the hand grips so that when the child grasps the supports, the elbow is slightly flexed, not straight.[6]	Allows for optimal use of the muscle groups needed for proper crutch walking.
5. Have the child stand with the crutches for several minutes until comfortable.	Allows the child to become familiar with the crutches and allows for adjustment.
6. Make sure that the child's pathway is clear of any obstacles.	Ensures that the child does not trip over any obstacles while learning to use the crutches.
7. Instruct the child to look forward and not at the feet when walking with the crutches.[6]	Helps the child to maintain balance by looking at the horizon. Also makes the child aware of upcoming obstacles.
8. Stand at one side of, and slightly behind, the child, with a hand supporting the child from behind.[6]	Helps the child to maintain balance and to prevent falls.
9. Teach the three-point gait (weight bearing or non–weight bearing).	The smaller child will maintain a better balance using the three-point gait.
10. Have the child lean slightly forward, bearing weight on the uninjured foot. Move both the crutches and the injured foot forward. Remind the child not to bear weight on the injured foot.[6]	
11. When the child has balanced his or her weight on both crutches, instruct the child to swing the uninjured foot forward to meet the crutches.[6] Teach the child not to swing the foot past the crutches.	Avoids causing a loss of balance and possible further injury.
12. Repeat Steps 10 and 11.	
13. Teach the child that crutches are not toys or weapons and should not be used by other children.	Prevents possible injury to other children.
14. Document that the child was in-	Communicates the nursing interven-

Table 9.3. (*cont.*)

NURSING ACTIONS	RATIONALE
structed on crutch walking, how the child was able to ambulate with the crutches, and whether the child was taught non–weight bearing or weight bearing.	tions and observations to health-care professionals.

The three most common casting materials used are plaster, fiberglass, and synthetic products. The plaster cast (Specialist™ plaster bandage) is made of open weave cotton rolls that are saturated with anhydrous calcium sulfate.[8] The fiberglass cast (Scotchcast™ casting tape) has the advantage of being lighter in weight and more durable.[8] The synthetic cast (delta-lite™ casting tape), also durable and lightweight, bonds to plaster for easy repair of plaster casts.[8]

Contraindications If the fracture site cannot be stabilized by casting (e.g., because of swelling), another form of immobilization should be considered.[3]

Complications Pressure sores on any bony prominence and decreased neuro-vascular function to the distal extremity due to increased swelling.[7]

Equipment

Casting material
  plaster
  fiberglass
  synthetic
Cast padding (Webril™)
Stockinette
Knife or scissors
Floor covering
Gloves
Sedatives or analgesics, if ordered
Lubricant jelly (to prevent fiberglass material from sticking to hands or gloves)
Plastic-lined pail of tepid water
Plaster trap in the sink
Alcohol wipes

Psychosocial Considerations For children who receive casts, many thoughts go through their minds. Children need to be told what they will feel during the casting process (soft, then warm, then cool and heavy). When possible, children should see a cast placed on a doll or stuffed animal prior to receiving their own casts and should be allowed to help with cast application if they show an interest in doing so. Offer children a choice of color or design of casting material, if they are available.

Children like to have their casts autographed by their friends and families. Children, as well as their parents, should be taught cast care. Parents can be present for casting, if they desire, to provide comfort and reassurance for the child.

Cast removal may also occur in the ED. The removal of a cast with an electric cast cutter is very noisy and frightening for the young child. Young children may have fears that the cast cutter will cut off their arm or leg. Children need to be told what they will hear and feel (loud buzzing noise, vibrations); they need reassurance that the cast cutter will not hurt their arm or leg.

Allowing the child to wear brightly colored ear muffs or to play music on a portable tape player with headphones during cast removal reduces the noise and decreases anxiety. If these devices are used, clean after each use.

Nursing responsibilities are described in Table 9.4.

Table 9.4.   Nursing Responsibilities

NURSING ACTIONS	RATIONALE
1. Explain the procedure to the child and the family.	Enhances their understanding and cooperation.
2. Assess the child's neurovascular status.	Provides a baseline neurovascular assessment.
3. Administer analgesic and sedative medications, as ordered by the physician, prior to casting.	Helps to relieve pain during the procedure.
4. Remove clothing and jewelry from the injured extremity.[7]	Avoids a constricting injury due to swelling.
5. Cover the floor and bedding with linen savers.	Prevents soiling of the floor and bedding with casting material.
6. Grasp the extremity properly to assist in cast application. **Arm:** Grasp the fingers and upper arm if necessary, off the side of the bed, to permit exposure of the entire arm. **Leg:** Grasp the toes in one hand, and hold the upper thigh with the other hand, and maintain flexion of the knee.	Helps to keep the injured extremity reduced and in the position of function during the casting procedure.
7. The physician places a stockinette or cast padding on the extremity. Ensure that extra padding is placed over bony prominences.	Helps to ensure that the padding is placed smoothly and snugly on the extremity. Prevents tissue breakdown at pressure points.
8. The physician submerges the casting material into water for approximately 1 minute, or until the bubbles no longer rise.	Activates the substance on the casting material so that the material may be molded to the extremity.
9. The physician squeezes the excess water out of the casting material.	The casting material dries faster if the excess water is expressed.
10. Starting at the distal end of the extremity, the physician smoothly wraps the casting material in an	Keeps the cast uniformly thick.

Table 9.4. (*cont.*)

NURSING ACTIONS	RATIONALE
overlapping manner toward the proximal end.	
11. As each layer of the casting material is placed, it is smoothed and rubbed in a circumferential and longitudinal direction.	Eliminates wrinkles and possible pressure points.[7] Makes a smooth, solid and well-fused cast.
12. The physician gently molds the casting material to the extremity.	Ensures that there are no pressure points; keeps the extremity from rotating.
13. *Always* use the palmar surface of the hands when handling the wet cast.[7]	Ensures that inadvertent pressure points are not created while handling the cast.
14. Reassess the child's neurovascular status, as well as the tightness of the cast.	Establishes that the cast was not applied too tightly and that the circulation is not impaired by its placement.
15. Tell the child that he or she may feel a radiation of warmth from the cast as the plaster begins to dry.	Heat is transmitted during the drying process.
16. Remove the casting residue from the skin, using alcohol wipes.	Keeps the skin from becoming irritated, which may lead to breakdown.
17. Elevate the casted extremity on a pillow; avoid indenting the wet plaster.	Helps to keep the swelling of the injured extremity at a minimum.
18. Obtain a postreduction x-ray of the casted extremity.	Ensures that the reduction of the fracture site was maintained.
19. Document how the child tolerated the procedure, the neurovascular status of the extremity before and after casting, and the instructions given to the child and parents about cast care.	Communicates the nursing interventions and observations to health-care professionals.
20. Teach the child and parents the importance of continuous evaluation of the cast and the distal extremity.	Allows for early identification of a potential problem.
a. Tell the child to report any increasing or unrelieved pain.	Pain may be an indication of an early pressure sore over a bony prominence.
b. Tell the parents and child to check for increased swelling of the toes or fingers.	If swelling continues, circulation may become impeded.
c. Tell the child and parent to check for capillary refill and color of the digits of the injured extremity.	Decreased capillary refill or a change in color of the digits from pink to blue is an indication that distal circulation is obstructed.

Table 9.4.   *(cont.)*

NURSING ACTIONS	RATIONALE
d. Tell the child and parent to check the fingers or toes for coolness, tingling, numbness, or decreased function, as well as to check for odor or discoloration coming from the cast.	A cool extremity may indicate decreased circulation to the extremity or neurovascular impairment. It also indicates that an ulceration has occurred or that an infection may be present.

ASSISTING WITH CLOSED REDUCTION

Indications   A closed reduction is indicated to bring fracture fragments into their anatomical position and alignment.[9] It is also used to reduce a dislocation. Manipulation and manual traction are used to perform the reduction.[9] A closed reduction may be performed either in the ED with local anesthesia and/or sedation or in the operating room under general anesthesia.

Contraindications   An open fracture, the possibility of neurovascular compromise.[10]

Complications   Incomplete reduction requiring open reduction.

Equipment

> Appropriate anesthesia or sedation
> > Bier block[10]
> > Demerol–Phenergan–Thorazine combination[11]
> > Fentanyl–Midazolam combination[11] doses:
> > Nitrous oxide (50%)[11]
> Traction device
> Appropriate postreduction immobilization
> > Casting material
> > Splints
> > Traction
> Cardiorespiratory monitor, automated BP monitor, resuscitation equipment

Psychosocial Considerations   The psychosocial considerations for a closed reduction are the same as for casting, with one exception. For the closed reduction, the child should receive sedation or analgesia. Children need to be told what they will feel and what will happen to them, even though they have been sedated. The parents may not want to be present during the reduction, because the manipulation of the extremity can appear distressing.

Nursing responsibilities are described in Table 9.5.

Table 9.5.   Nursing Responsibilities

NURSING ACTIONS	RATIONALE
1. Explain to the child and the family the need for the closed reduction.	Enhances their understanding and cooperation.
2. Assess the child's neurovascular status.	If the neurovascular status is not intact, a closed reduction is inappropriate.
3. Medicate the child according to the	Helps to relax the extremity muscles

Table 9.5. *(cont.)*

NURSING ACTIONS	RATIONALE
physician's order. Attach to the child the cardiorespiratory and blood pressure monitors. Have appropriate resuscitation equipment and Narcan (Naloxone) readily available.	and to sedate the child. Both are very important in making the manipulation less traumatic and easier to accomplish.
4. Remove all clothing and jewelry from the injured extremity.[7]	Reduces the possibility of a constricting injury due to swelling and enables complete visualization of the extremity.
5. Assist the physician with manual traction of the extremity, as appropriate.	
6. Reassess the child's neurovascular status.	Ensures that the reduction did not impair the neurovascular function of the extremity. If impairment is noted, then an open reduction may be necessary.
7. Assist in maintaining postreduction stabilization (see Table 9.4).	Prevents the fracture from becoming misaligned.
8. Assist in obtaining postreduction x-rays.	
9. Document the sedation medication given to the child, how the child tolerated the procedure, the neurovascular status of the extremity before and after the reduction, and what child and parents were taught about cast care. Document the child's level of consciousness upon discharge.	Communicates the nursing interventions and observations to health-care professionals.
10. Teach the child and parents the importance of continuous evaluation of the cast and the distal extremity.	The child and the parents will be able to indicate a potential problem early.
a. Tell the child to report any increasing or unrelieved pain.	Pain may be an indication of an early pressure sore over a bony prominence.
b. Tell the parent and the child to check for increased swelling of the toes or fingers.	If swelling continues, circulation may become impeded.
c. Tell the child and parents to check for capillary refill and color of the digits of the injured extremity.	Decreased capillary refill or a change in color of the digits from pink to blue is an indication that distal circulation is obstructed.
d. Tell the child and parents to check the fingers or toes for coolness, tingling, numbness, or decreased function, as well as to check for odor or discoloration coming from the cast.	A cool extremity may indicate decreased circulation to the extremity or neurovascular impairment. It may also indicate that an ulceration has occurred or that an infection may be present.

REFERENCES

1. Hilt N, Schmitt W. Pediatric orthopedic nursing. St. Louis: C.V. Mosby, 1975:11.
2. Rourke K, Phelan A, Miller M. Orthopedic emergencies. In: Kelley S, ed. Pediatric emergency nursing. Norwalk, CT: Appleton & Lange, 1988:418.
3. Browne PS. Basic facts of fractures. 2nd ed. London: Blackwell Scientific, 1988:10.
4. Caroline NL. Emergency care in the streets. 4th ed. Boston: Little, Brown, 1991:377–380.
5. Grant H, Murray R, Bergeron J. Emergency care. 5th ed. Englewood Cliffs, NJ: Brady–Prentice-Hall, 1990:257–259.
6. Jackson EW. Nursing '82 books: Nursing photo series. Providing early mobility. Springhouse, PA: Intermed Communications, 1982:104, 109–110.
7. Lourie J, Bradlow A, Sutters M. Essentials of accident and emergency care. London: Churchill Livingstone, 1987:104.
8. Jackson EW. Nursing '82 books: Nursing photo series. Working with orthopedic patients. Springhouse, PA: Intermed Communications, 1982:59.
9. Suddarth DS. The Lippincott manual of nursing practice. 5th ed. Philadelphia: J.B. Lippincott, 1991:768.
10. Mayeda DV. Orthopedic injuries. In: Barkin R, Rosen P. Emergency pediatrics. A guide to ambulatory care. 3rd ed. St. Louis: C.V. Mosby, 1990:419.
11. Greene MG. The Harriet Lane handbook. 12th ed. St. Louis: Mosby-Year Book 1991:261.

CHAPTER 10

Procedures Involving the Integumentary System

Kathy MacPherson

OVERVIEW OF PEDIATRIC DIFFERENCES IN THE INTEGUMENTARY SYSTEM

As the largest organ of the body, the integumentary system protects the internal structures, regulates the body temperature, senses the environment, regulates fat storage and metabolism, and regulates water and salt metabolism via perspiration. Skin thickness generally is less in infants and children. On persons of all ages, the thickness of the epidermis varies, being thinnest on the eyelids; genitalia; anterior neck; flexor surfaces of the arms and forearms; and the antecubital, popliteal, and interdigital spaces. The skin is the thickest on the palms, soles, and scalp.[1]

Because of their larger ratio of body surface area to weight, children are at risk for hypothermia. Children lose more heat from evaporation and convexion, as compared to adults. In addition, cold-stressed neonates and infants less than 6 months of age are unable to shiver to generate body heat, so they must break down brown fat to maintain their body temperature.[2]

The thermoregulatory needs of children receiving treatment in the emergency department (ED) must be met. During trauma resuscitation, cover the child with warm blankets after the primary and secondary trauma surveys are completed. Additional heat sources should be available (e.g., external heat lamps, blood/fluid warmers).

Throughout childhood, skin lesions of various etiologies occur, such as dermatitis and scalded-skin syndrome. A careful assessment of the skin provides much information about the child's health status and should be included in every physical examination.

WOUND CARE

Indications   Wounds are cleaned and debrided to promote healing and to prevent infection.

Contraindications   None.

Complications   Allergy to skin-cleansing solutions, to antiseptic ointment, or to adhesive tape, which may cause skin redness, rash, or excoriation.[3] Ingestion of the antiseptic ointment if the wound is poorly bandaged.

Equipment

> Irrigation solution
> Antiseptic solution/ointment
> Sterile forceps and probe
> Sterile gloves
> Analgesics, if ordered by physician
> Sterile bowl
> Papoose board
> Goggles, if needed
> Irrigation syringe or commercially prepared irrigation set
> Dressing materials: sterile gauze pads, antiseptic ointment, tape or roller gauze

Psychosocial Considerations   Wound care can be uncomfortable for the child, not only in terms of pain, but also in being positioned and secured for the procedure. Young children may believe they are being punished for their injury. Distraction techniques or sedation must be considered for a lengthy procedure. Parents can be present if they choose, so that they can learn how to do the wound care at home.

Nursing responsibilities are described in Table 10.1.

Table 10.1.   Nursing Responsibilities

NURSING ACTIONS	RATIONALE
1. Explain to the child and the family the need for the wound care. Ask whether the child has any allergies to the antiseptic solutions or medications that will be used. Assess the child's immunization status.	Enhances their understanding and cooperation. Avoids allergic reactions. Ensures an adequate immunization status. If an animal bite occurred, inquire about the animal's rabies status.
2. Place the equipment on a clean overbed tray or table at the child's bedside.	Having a clean area prevents potential contamination.
3. Position the child for the procedure; drape the area and expose the site to be dressed. Cover the child with a gown or sheet. With infants and young children, a papoose board may be necessary to ensure proper application of dressings. (See Chapter 3, Positioning and Securing Children for Procedures.)	Prevents cross-contamination.
4. Don sterile gloves and goggles, if needed.	Decreases chance of wound contamination; complies with universal precautions.

Table 10.1.   *(cont.)*

NURSING ACTIONS	RATIONALE
5. Prepare the area to be cleaned.	Prevents infection; promotes wound healing.
Sutured Wounds	
a. Apply antiseptic ointment and a bandage or sterile gauze sponges.	
b. Secure with tape, roller gauze or Ace bandages. (See Table 10.4.)	
Nonsutured wounds	
a. Saturate gauze sponges with antiseptic solution.	
b. Fold the saturated sponges and grasp one with sterile forceps. Clean the area by moving the soaked sponge in a circle, starting at the center of the wound and enlarging the circle to the outer edges.	The presence of bacteria is lower at the center of the injury and greatest at the outer edges.[3]
c. For infected or extremely dirty wounds, don goggles and irrigate the wound with copious amounts of saline using a syringe or a commercially available irrigation set.	Lavage lowers the bacterial count and potentially lessens the amount of foreign material or devitalized tissue in the wound.[4]
d. Rinse the area with normal saline, if necessary, and dry well with gauze sponges.	The skin must be dry for the dressing to remain intact.
e. Apply ointment and bandages.	
6. Administer tetanus prophylaxis, if needed; if rabies is suspected, set up a schedule to begin treatment.	Ensures adequate tetanus and rabies prophylaxis.
7. Release the child from the papoose board (if used). Praise the child for being cooperative.	Allows the child to be mobile. Promotes a sense of mastery.
8. Explain the wound care to the child and family. Teach them the signs of wound infection.	
9. Clean the instruments and discard the gloves.	
10. Document the appearance of the wound, the type of antiseptic solution used, the kind of dressing applied, and the instructions given to the parents.	Communicates the nursing interventions and observations to health-care professionals.

ASSISTING WITH SUTURING

Indications   Suturing is a method of approximating the torn edges of tissue with suture material, such as silk, chromic, staples, or synthetic material (absorbable or nonabsorbable). Suturing a wound promotes healing and minimizes tissue scarring. The decision to leave a wound open for a short period of time or until complete healing has occurred is largely based on concerns about secondary wound infection with a primary closure.

Contraindications   Suturing is often not attempted with (1) animal bites, (2) human bites, (3) lacerations that are contaminated, and (4) lacerations that occurred more than 8 hours before the child is brought to the emergency department.

Complications   Infection of the wound due to inadequate cleaning; allergy to local anesthetic, skin cleansing solution, or adhesive tape, which may cause skin redness, rash or excoriation.[3]

Equipment

> Commercially prepared suture kit
> Suture material
> Antiseptic solution
> Sterile gloves
> Disposable razor, if needed
> Irrigating solution
> Irrigation syringe or commercially prepared irrigation set
> Dressing materials: sterile gauze pads, antiseptic ointment, tape, or roller gauze
> Papoose board, if needed
> Local anesthetic (0.5%, 1% or 2% lidocaine with or without epinephrine; TAC—tetracaine, adrenalin [epinephrine], cocaine)
> Syringe and needle to inject local anesthetic
> Gloves, goggles (if needed)

Note   Local anesthetics containing epinephrine are not used on highly contaminated wounds or fingers, toes, ears, nose, or penis because of their vasoconstrictive effect.

Psychosocial Considerations   This procedure is distressing to children because they are restrained and uncomfortable. Young children may believe they are being punished for a real or imagined wrongdoing. Talk to children throughout the procedure and tell them what they will feel (cool soap, pinching, etc.). Allow them to cry and to move other body parts that do not need restraint (e.g., toes, feet) during the procedure. Parents can be present if they choose, but they should not be asked to restrain their child or to stay in the room if they are uncomfortable in doing so (see Figure 10.1).

Several factors must be considered when the child returns for suture removal. The child may remember the suturing process and may become distressed upon seeing the suture room. If the suturing experience was a negative one, where the child required restraint for a prolonged period of time, this distress may be heightened.

Prepare the suture removal equipment immediately before the procedure

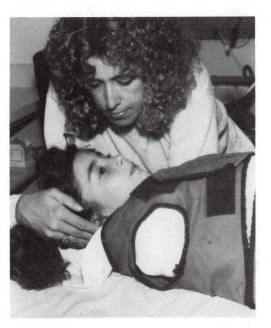

Figure 10.1.   The presence of a parent during suturing can provide distraction and comfort for the child.

to avoid causing undue distress. The child may require the papoose board, or sedation, relative to the type of repair.

Parents should be instructed about skin care following suture removal, especially the use of sunscreen on the face to prevent scarring.

Nursing responsibilities are described in Table 10.2.

Table 10.2.   Nursing Responsibilities

NURSING ACTIONS	RATIONALE
1. Explain to the child and the family the need for the suturing. Assess the child's immunization status. Ask whether the child has any allergies to antiseptic solutions or medications that will be used.	Enhances their understanding and cooperation. Avoids allergic reactions. Ensures an adequate immunization status.
2. Place the equipment on a clean over-bed tray or table at the child's bedside. Avoid reaching across the sterile field or the wound during the procedure.	Helps to prevent possible contamination.
3. Position the child for the procedure; the papoose board may be necessary.	Prevents unnecessary movement during the procedure and decreases the chance of further injury.
4. Provide privacy by closing the treatment room door and covering the child. Adjust the overhead light as necessary.	Shows respect for the child. Allows maximum visibility of the wound.

Table 10.2. *(cont.)*

NURSING ACTIONS	RATIONALE
5. Don sterile gloves, and goggles (if needed).	Decreases chance of wound contamination; complies with universal precautions.
6. Clean and irrigate the area to be repaired with antiseptic solution, and rinse it well (or assist the physician in doing so). Shave hair if necessary (but never shave eyebrows). Clean the area in a circular motion away from the area to be sutured.	Reduces the risk of infection with skin organisms.
7. Cover the area with sterile gauze pad.	Prevents contamination from airborne organisms.
8. Prepare the child for injection of the local anesthetic or application of TAC.	Informs the child of what to expect and eliminates surprises.
a. **Local anesthetic**—tell the child that she or he will feel a "pinch and a burn."	
b. **TAC**—Place the TAC, in the prescribed amount, on a 2 × 2 gauze pad, and apply it to the laceration with a gloved hand, using direct pressure for approximately 20 minutes.	
9. Assist, as needed, throughout the procedure; help the child to cope by using distraction, storytelling, imagery, and so on. Suggest sedation if the child is not able to tolerate the procedure.	
10. Apply the antiseptic ointment and bandage appropriately (see Tables 10.1 and 10.4).	
11. Administer tetanus prophylaxis, if needed. Release the child from the papoose board and praise her or him for cooperating.	
12. Document the number of sutures and how the child tolerated the procedure. Ensure the family's understanding of the wound care follow-up instructions. Instruct the child and family regarding what to look for in the event of wound infection, such as fever, redness, swelling, or drainage from the suture site. Ensure that the family knows when to return for suture removal.	Communicates the nursing interventions and observations to health-care professionals.

CARE OF MINOR BURNS (< 10% total body surface area)

Indications   Burns are an injury to body tissues caused by thermal, electrical, chemical, or radiant agents. The extent of the injury is determined by the amount of tissue exposed to the agent, the time and duration of the exposure, and by the nature of the agent. The treatment of burns includes pain relief, careful asepsis, prevention of infection, maintenance of the balance of fluids and electrolytes, and good nutrition.[7]

Contraindications   None.

Complications   Infection, allergic reaction to the analgesia or to the topical antimicrobial agent.

Equipment

>   Analgesia, as ordered
>   Sterile gloves
>   Normal saline solution
>   Mild antiseptic solution
>   Sterile scissors, tissue forceps
>   Sterile cotton-tipped applicators
>   Sterile basins
>   Dressing materials: sterile gauze pads, topical antimicrobial agent, tape or roller
>   gauze

Psychosocial Considerations   Experiencing a minor burn injury is terrifying and very painful. The child may feel guilty if he or she caused the injury (e.g., playing with matches or firecrackers), or the child may be frightened by the repercussions from her or his parents for disobeying them. The young child who pulls a hot teacup onto her- or himself or who bites a plugged-in electrical cord will be very frightened, not only from the pain, but also from his or her parents' fearful reactions.

Parents may feel guilty if they believe they did not supervise the younger child properly. They may also fear that their child will be physically scarred from the injury.

Both the parents and the child need reassurance and comfort that everything possible is being done to help the child. The parents may not want to look at the injury and may choose to leave during the burn care and dressing change. Be supportive of their need to do this, and try to have one nurse support the child. Relaxation, distraction techniques, and analgesia should be employed. With minor burns, the child may want to remove her or his own dressings, as this gives the child a sense of control. However, children should not be forced to look at their burn injury; they will view it when they are psychologically ready to do so.

Parents must be taught how to care for the burn wound at home. If they do not appear comfortable performing wound care, either have them return to the ED for dressing changes, or have social services personnel arrange for a visiting nurse to come to the home. Counseling may be required for the child and the family, based on the circumstances surrounding the injury and their response to the injury.

Nursing responsibilities are described in Table 10.3.

Table 10.3. Nursing Responsibilities

NURSING ACTIONS	RATIONALE
1. Explain to the child and the family the need for burn care. Ask whether the child has any allergies to the antiseptic solution or medications that will be used. Assess the child's immunization status.	Enhances their understanding and cooperation. Avoids allergic reactions. Ensures an adequate immunization status.
2. Ensure adequate illumination of the treatment area. Open the supplies, using sterile technique, and arrange the items, in order of use, on a sterile field.	
3. Keep the room temperature warm by (a) using an overhead warmer, or (b) turning up the temperature in the room. If the room cannot be warmed, (a) expose the child as little as possible, and (b) wrap the child in warm blankets.	With large burns, body heat is lost, causing chilling.[5]
4. Assess the percentage, location, and depth of the burn, using a Lund & Browder chart; for subsequent treatment, assess for eschar separation, inflammation, purulent drainage, and the condition of the blisters.	Indicates possible infection or poor wound healing.
5. Administer analgesics as ordered by the physician. Acetaminophen or codeine or meperidine may be administered in small doses orally.	Minimizes pain.
6. Don gloves. Gently clean the burn wound with gauze sponges moistened with a mild antiseptic solution and normal saline.	Prevents wound contamination.
7. Carefully debride all loose tissue with sterile forceps and scissors. Observe for bleeding.	Reduces infection and allows the burn wound to begin the healing process. Bleeding indicates viable tissue.
8. Gently clean the area with saline solution.	Removes all loose tissue and the cleansing agent.
9. Change gloves before applying the dressing if the wound is to be dressed.	Prevents recontamination of the wound.
10. Thickly apply a topical antimicrobial agent to 4 × 4 gauze sponges. Cover the wound with the saturated sponges, being careful to cover all burned areas.	Promotes wound healing.

Table 10.3.   (*cont.*)

NURSING ACTIONS	RATIONALE
11. Wrap the bandages securely enough to stimulate circulation yet prevent constriction. (See Table 10.4.)	Allows for regrowth of the vascular bed. Increases the child's comfort.
12. Administer tetanus prophylaxis, if needed.	
13. Record the time, treatment, and pertinent wound observations after the burn is dressed. Note any comfort measures used and how the child tolerated the procedure.	Communicates the nursing interventions and observations to health-care professionals.
14. Teach the parents how to apply the dressings at home. Instruct them on how to observe for signs of infection, and give them a phone number to call if problems arise.	Decreases the potential for infection; ensures that the burn care will be completed.

BANDAGING

Indications   Bandages are designed to protect wounds from contamination and trauma. They provide compression, keep the wound sites dry, and immobilize the wound. Bandages also promote comfort by reducing exposure of the area to external stimuli (air, water, heat).

Contraindications   None. However, bandages may not be needed on some types of wounds, depending on physician preference or nursing judgment.

Complications   Bandages wrapped too tightly may impede circulation and cause tissue damage; bandages wrapped too loosely may not afford protection from infection and may adversely affect the healing process. A bandage that can be easily removed by the child may cause unintentional ingestion of the antiseptic ointment.

Equipment and Supplies

> Scissors
> Sterile forceps and probe
> Sterile gloves
> Tape
> Gauze sponges
> Ace wraps
> Roller gauze
> Band-Aid™s
> Analgesics, if ordered by physician
> Papoose board

Psychosocial Considerations   Bandaging a young child's wound is very challenging. Even if the wound does not require a bandage, the preschooler may appreciate a light bandage or a Band-Aid™. Avoid using the term *dressing,* as the young child may equate *dressing* with *salad dressing* instead of a bandage. Always explain to the child what he or she will feel during the procedure. When possible, allow the child to participate in the bandaging process by holding the bandage, tape, and so on. Have the parent place the bandage or have the parent return for a bandage change to ensure that they are changed properly.

Nursing responsibilities are described in Tables 10.4 through 10.8.

Table 10.4.   Nursing Responsibilities

NURSING ACTIONS	RATIONALE
1. Explain to the child and the family the need for the bandage.	Enhances their understanding and cooperation.
2. Place the equipment on a clean over-bed tray or table.	Prevents potential contamination.
3. Wash your hands.	Prevents spread of infection.
4. Position the child for the procedure, and drape the area to expose the site to be dressed. Cover the child with a gown or sheet. With infants and young children, a papoose board may be necessary, to ensure proper application of dressings (see Chapter 2).	Prevents cross-contamination.
5. Open and don the sterile gloves.	
6. Ensure that the area to be bandaged has had proper wound care.	
7. Follow the procedures listed in Tables 10.5, 10.6, 10.7, and 10.8, regarding bandaging in different areas of the body.	

Table 10.5.   Bandages for the Torso

NURSING ACTIONS	RATIONALE
1. Apply the medication as ordered, and cover the area with either 4 × 4 sponges or large (5 × 9) absorbent gauze pads.	
2. Wrap the area with sterile roller gauze, of the appropriate diameter for the child's size. Circle the chest/back area, and wrap around the clavicle areas (see Figure 10.2).	

Table 10.5.   *(cont.)*

NURSING ACTIONS	RATIONALE

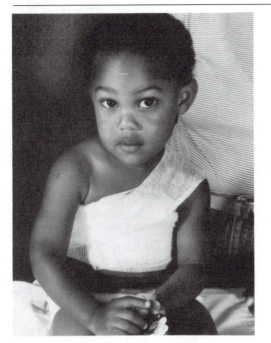

Figure 10.2. Securing a chest bandage by wrapping the roller gauze over a shoulder; both shoulders could also be covered in a figure-8, to secure the bandage.

3. Apply tape over the gauze in areas where the child can lift or scratch through the gauze.	Helps keep the bandage in place.
4. Another option is to use tube gauze or Flex-inet™. Measure the material to the size of the child's torso, and cut it at the appropriate length. Slip it over the child's head and arms.	
5. A clean white undershirt of the correct size would also hold the bandages in place and may be more comfortable for the child.	
6. Demonstrate the bandaging procedure to the child and the family, or have the parent perform the procedure prior to leaving the ED.	Ensures understanding of the bandaging process.
7. Clean the instruments and dispose of the gloves.	Prevents contamination of staff and other patients.
8. Document the kind of bandage applied and instructions given to the parents.	Communicates the nursing interventions and observations to health-care professionals.

Table 10.6. Bandages for Fingers and Toes

NURSING ACTIONS	RATIONALE
1. Assess neurovascular status. Wrap each digit separately with a 2 × 2 gauze pad.	Provides a baseline neurovascular assessment. Avoids adhering of digits during the healing process.
2. Wrap the appropriate size of roller gauze around the digit.	
3. Encircle the wrist or ankle with the bandage, and secure it with tape.	Prevents slippage of the bandage.
4. Another option is to use tube gauze.	
5. Demonstrate the bandaging procedure to the child and the family, or have the parent perform the procedure prior to leaving the ED.	Ensures understanding of the bandaging process.
6. Clean the instruments and dispose of the gloves; reassess neurovascular status.	Prevents contamination of staff and other patients; ensures that placement of the bandage did not impair neurovascular functioning.
7. Document the kind of bandage applied and the instructions given to the parents.	Communicates the nursing interventions and observations to health-care professionals.

Table 10.7. Dressings for Thighs and Buttocks

NURSING ACTIONS	RATIONALE
1. Apply 4 × 4 sponges.	
2. Use roller gauze in a figure-8 pattern over the wound, bringing it up to encircle the waist.	
3. After encircling the waist, the roller gauze is brought back down to the thigh area.	
4. The end of the roller gauze may be slit, in order to tie it into a knot, and then reinforced with tape.	
5. Demonstrate the bandaging procedure to the child and the family, or have the parent perform the procedure prior to leaving the ED.	Ensures understanding of the bandaging process.
6. Clean the instruments and dispose of the gloves.	Prevents contamination of staff and other patients.
7. Document the kind of bandage applied and the instructions given to the parents.	Communicates the nursing interventions and observations to health-care professionals.

Table 10.8. Bandages for the Upper Arm and Shoulder Area

NURSING ACTIONS	RATIONALE
1. Apply 4 × 4 sponges.	
2. Use roller gauze in a figure-8 pattern over the wound, and bring it around to encircle the clavicle area or around the chest area.	
3. The end of the roller gauze may be slit, in order to tie it into a knot, and then reinforced with tape.	
4. The knotted roller gauze should not be too tight to afford better stability. Bandages can be reinforced with tape.	Avoids impairment of circulation.
5. Demonstrate the bandaging procedure to the child and the family, or have the parent perform the procedure prior to leaving the ED.	Assures understanding of bandaging process.
6. Clean the instruments and dispose of the gloves.	Prevents contamination of staff and other patients.
7. Document the kind of bandage applied and the instructions given to the parents.	Communicates the nursing interventions and observations to health-care professionals.

CARE OF AMPUTATED BODY PARTS

Indications   Preservation of both the amputated body part and the stump are required if replantation is to be undertaken.

Contraindications   The physician should decide whether replantation is possible, depending on the extent of the child's injury and the viability of the amputated part. Replantation usually will not be attempted if the child has other major trauma or crush injuries.[7]

Complications   Loss of blood, ischemia, and irreversible tissue damage within 6 hours if the amputated part is not kept cold.

Equipment

 Sterile gloves
 Normal saline or lactated Ringer's solution
 Sterile gauze
 Sterile towel
 Airtight bags or containers, of various sizes
 Ice
 Labels
 Analgesics, if ordered by physician

Psychosocial Considerations   Experiencing an amputation is extremely devastating for the child, the family, and the ED staff. The child should be protected from viewing mutilating injuries. The child's head can be turned away during the examination of the stump. Avoid talking about how "horrible" the injury is, as this will only heighten the child's distress and fears. Seeing the amputated part itself is very individualized, and if it occurs, it should only be after consultation with experienced pediatric health care professionals.

The parents need to be told by the physician honestly but tactfully what the chances are for replantation. They should be allowed to touch and to talk with the child as soon as possible. Counseling is essential for the child who experiences an amputation, whether or not the body part is replanted.

Nursing responsibilities are described in Table 10.9.

Table 10.9. Nursing Responsibilities

NURSING ACTIONS	RATIONALE
1. Explain to the child and the family the plan of care. Reassure them that everything is being done to help the child. Ask about the child's immunization status. Consider administering analgesics.	Helps the child and family to trust the staff; allows for reasonable expectations. Ensures an adequate immunization status. Decreases pain and discomfort.
2. Don sterile gloves; flush the amputated part with normal saline or lactated Ringer's solution. Rinse off debris, and keep the exposed end moist. Do not scrub or debride the part.	Avoids further trauma and tissue damage.
3. Gently pat dry the amputated part with sterile gauze, then wrap the part in saline-soaked sterile gauze. Wrap the gauze with a sterile towel. Put the wrapped part in a watertight container or bag with the child's name and hospital identification number.[7] *Do not* place the amputated part directly in ice or ice water.	Decreases irreversible tissue and blood vessel damage. Direct placement of the amputated part in ice or ice water will cause tissue damage.
4. Place the part, in its watertight container, inside a large bag or container filled with ice water. Seal the bag or container. Keep the bag cold until the time for replantation. Always protect the part from direct contact with ice. *Never* use dry ice.	Dry ice is too cold and can cause irreversible tissue damage, making the part unsuitable for replantation.
5. Label the bag with the child's name, date, and hospital identification number; the time of amputation, the time when the cooling process started, and identification of ampu-	Prevents accidental discarding or opening. Communicates the nursing interventions and observations to health-care professionals.

Table 10.9.   *(cont.)*

NURSING ACTIONS	RATIONALE
tated part. Document this information on child's ED record.	
6. Clean the stump from which the amputation occurred, using sterile gloves, then flush the injured area of the stump with normal saline or lactated Ringer's solution. Do not scrub or debride the area. After rinsing, wrap the area in saline-soaked gauze and a sterile towel.	Prevents infection. Prevents tissue and blood vessel damage.
7. Administer tetanus immunization, if needed.	
8. Document the appearance of the stump, the amount of bleeding, and the presence of pulses, sensation, color, movement, or pain; also note whether tetanus prophylaxis or analgesics were administered.	Communicates the nursing interventions and observations to health-care professionals.

MEASURES TO MAINTAIN BODY TEMPERATURE

Indications   The body temperature in healthy individuals is regulated within narrow limits. Intervention may be indicated when the body temperature rises above normal (hyperthermia) or falls below normal (hypothermia). Cooling is used to treat hyperthermic conditions, such as fever, heat exhaustion, and heat stroke. Cooling measures are *not* routinely needed for the treatment of fever in children but are reserved for cases in which the fever is adversely affecting the child, and treatment with an antipyretic (e.g., acetaminophen) is ineffective. Rewarming is used in such conditions as drowning, frostbite, and trauma.

Contraindications   None known.

Complications

Cooling   Cooling of the child is done gradually to prevent arrhythmias and to reduce shivering, which in turn can cause the body's core temperature to rise.[8]

Warming   Methods of rewarming children can cause early warming of the skin and extremities, with peripheral vasodilation, resulting in shunting of cold, acidemic blood to the central circulation[8] and loss of heat.

Equipment

For Cooling

> Basin/tub of tepid (not cold) water
> Thermometer

Towels/washcloths
Linen-saver pads
Clean clothing (to be used after bath)
Hyperthermia blanket
Bath tub toys or items to help occupy the child

For Warming

Overhead warmer
Aquamatic K-pad, distilled water
Chemical hot pack
Thermometer
Blankets
Hypothermia blanket

Psychosocial Considerations   Children and adolescents who have had heat stroke may have permanently impaired heat tolerance;[8] they should be taught how to prevent future heat-related illnesses.

For the hypothermic child, constant reassurance and explanations are necessary to keep the child from becoming more distressed. Explain to the parent why these measures are being undertaken to help decrease their anxiety.

Nursing responsibilities are described in Tables 10.10 through 10.14.

Table 10.10.   Nursing Responsibilities—Cooling

NURSING ACTIONS	RATIONALE
1. Explain to the child and the family the need for hypothermic measures and provide privacy. Make sure the room is free of drafts.	Enhances their understanding and cooperation; shows respect for the child's needs. Reduces potential for chilling.
2. Assess the child's general condition.	The child's condition affects his or her response to treatment.
3. Wash your hands. Measure and document the child's temperature and other vital signs.	Provides baseline information.
4. Remove the child's clothes, and cover her or him with a towel. Put the linen-saver pad under the child if cooling is carried out on the child's bed. If the child is sponged in a tub, the pad is not needed.	Prevents the bedding from becoming wet and causing chilling.
5. If using a hypothermia blanket, follow the manufacturer's directions.	Allows for proper application and prevents injury to the child.
6. Alternative cooling methods are as follows:	
a. For heat stroke, massage the child's skin with ice, keep the	These measures increase convection and evaporative heat loss.[8]

Table 10.10.   (*cont.*)

NURSING ACTIONS	RATIONALE
child's skin moist, and direct fans onto the child.[8]	
b. Monitor the child's temperature, and discontinue cooling when the rectal temperature falls to approximately 38.5°C.[8]	
7. Observe the child for chilling, shivering, pallor, mottling, cyanosis of lips and nailbeds.	If any of these are observed, the cooling process is too rapid. Discontinue it, and cover the child with a sheet.
8. Document the child's condition, vital signs, duration of cooling treatment, and the child's response to treatment.	Communicates the nursing interventions and observations to health-care professionals.

Table 10.11.   Nursing Responsibilities—Warming

NURSING ACTIONS	RATIONALE
1. Explain to the child and the family the need for the hyperthermic measures.	Enhances their understanding and cooperation.
2. Assess the child's condition; check the physician's orders for the preferred type of warming device.	Provides a baseline assessment.
3. Provide privacy, and make sure the room is free of drafts.	Promotes effective warming.
4. Monitor the child's temperature throughout the warming process. Ensure adequacy of ventilation and circulation.	Measures the effectiveness of the procedure.
5. Active rewarming techniques are either external or core.[8] *External* techniques include electric blankets, hot water bottles, overhead warmers, thermal mattresses and warm water baths.[8]	Use with caution to prevent complications associated with rewarming.
Core techniques include peritoneal dialysis, inhalation rewarming, hemodialysis, extra-corporeal blood rewarming, and mediastinal irrigation.[8] These technique are used with severe hypothermia (temperature less than 32°C).[8]	Quicker effectiveness and decreased chance of an afterdrop in temperature, dysrhythmias, or significant hypotension.[8]

Table 10.12. Method for External Rewarming

NURSING ACTIONS	RATIONALE
1. Before putting the child on the K-pad or under the warmer, check the heat being generated.	Prevents burning of the child and tests the heat distribution.
2. Apply the heat-generating source for the prescribed amount of time. Protect the child from the heat source with a light layer of linen between the skin and the heat-generating source. Heating pads should not be used on infants and young children.	
3. Assess the child's skin condition and general condition.	
4. Continue treatment for 20–30 minutes, or as ordered by physician.	Allows for proper rewarming.
5. Remove the child from the warming device if the child reports pain or discomfort or if there is increased pallor, swelling, or redness.	The rewarming process is too rapid.
6. Cover the child with blankets, and assess the temperature and vital signs.	Determines the effectiveness of the treatment and allows for a comparison with the baseline.
7. Document the vital signs before and after rewarming and the child's response to the treatment.	Communicates the nursing interventions and observations to health-care professionals.

REFERENCES
1. Wagner M, ed. Care of the burn-injured patient: Multidisciplinary involvement. Littleton, MA: PSG Publishing, 1981;10.
2. Hazinski MF. Children are different. In: Hazinski MF, ed. Nursing care of the critically ill child. 2nd ed. St. Louis: Mosby-Yearbook 1992;4.
3. Donahue S, Felice P, Wind S. Physical treatments: Wound care. In: Procedures. Springhouse, PA: Springhouse Corp., 1985;244;241.
4. Templeton JM, Ziegler MM. Minor trauma and minor lesions. In: Fleisher G, Ludwig S, eds. Textbook of pediatric emergency medicine. 2nd ed. Baltimore: Williams & Wilkins, 1988:923.
5. Templeton J, Broennle AM. Emergency department anesthetic management. In: Fleisher G, Ludwig S, eds. Textbook of pediatric emergency medicine. 2nd ed. Baltimore: Williams & Wilkins, 1988;65.
6. Whitaker L. Plastic surgical emergencies: Facial injuries and burns. In: Fleisher G, Ludwig S, eds. Textbook of pediatric emergency medicine. 2nd ed. Baltimore: Williams & Wilkins, 1988;1058.
7. Anonymous. Musculoskeletal emergencies: What to do first. In: Emergencies. Springhouse, PA: Springhouse Corp., 1985;346,345,350.

8. Thompson A. Environmental emergencies. In: Fleisher G, Ludwig S, eds. Textbook of pediatric emergency medicine. 2nd ed. Baltimore: Williams & Wilkins, 1988;611;612;615.

11

Eye, Ear, Nose, and Oral Procedures

Lisa M. *Bernardo* and Marianne Bove

EYE IRRIGATION

Indications Eye irrigation is indicated to remove loose debris and foreign bodies[1] or to dilute or remove irritants or chemicals as indicated by poison-control recommendations.

Contraindications As indicated by poison control recommendations; evidence of penetrating eye trauma.

Complications Injury to eye tissues.

Equipment

> Soft rubber bulb syringe or irrigation tubing
> Warmed normal saline solution
> Towels or linen-saver pads
> Topical proparacaine (0.5%) or other topical anesthetic
> Papoose board (if needed)
> Emesis basin
> Eye patch (if indicated)
> Gloves

Psychosocial Considerations Young children may become frightened by being secured and they may believe this treatment is punishment for getting chemicals or materials into their eyes. Older children may be able to understand why the irrigation is necessary and therefore should be able to cooperate.

Parents should be permitted to remain with the child to comfort and distract him or her during the procedure. However, they may not wish to be present and should be permitted to leave the room if they are more comfortable in doing so.

Nursing responsibilities are described in Table 11.1.

Table 11.1. Nursing Responsibilities

NURSING ACTIONS	RATIONALE
1. Explain to the child and the family the need for the eye irrigation.	Enhances their understanding and cooperation.
2. Assemble the equipment.	Hastens the efficiency of the procedure.
3. Wash your hands.	
4. Secure the child on a papoose board (see Chapter 3).	Prevents injury during procedure.
5. Place towels under the child's head; place an emesis basin on the side of the head that will be irrigated.	Collects excess irrigating solution.
6. Administer topical proparacaine (0.5%) to the affected eye(s), as ordered by the physician.	Decreases blepharospasm; allows for thorough irrigation of both conjunctival sacs.[2]
7. Using the bulb syringe or irrigation tubing, gently direct a stream of warm irrigating solution into the lower fornix, working from the medial canthus outward. Instruct the child to look up or straight ahead.	Allows for proper irrigation of eye.
8. Use the amount of solution recommended by the regional poison control center; however 2 liters of saline is generally optimal.[2,3]	Ensures adequate irrigation of eyes.
9. Alternatively, continuous irrigation can be obtained with scleral contact lenses.[3] Refer to the manufacturer's instructions for their proper use.	
10. Dry the child's face. Release the child from the securing device and praise the child for cooperating. Encourage the parent to comfort the child.	Provides a sense of control and mastery.
11. Wash your hands.	Prevents contamination.
12. Apply an eye patch or shield (see Tables 11.3 and 11.4).	
13. Document the length of time for the procedure, the amount and type of solution used, characteristics of the irrigated solution, and how the child tolerated the procedure.	Communicates the nursing interventions and observations to other health-care professionals.

PLACEMENT OF AN EYE PATCH OR EYE SHIELD

Indications   An eye patch, which keeps the lid closed with gentle pressure, is used for treatment of corneal abrasions.[2] In contrast, for blunt eye trauma, a perforated metal or plastic eye shield, which does not apply pressure to the globe, is used, to prevent further damage to the eye.[2]

Contraindications   An eye patch is not used with ocular trauma, as this may increase intraocular pressure.

Complications   Increased intraocular pressure from the application of an eye patch.

Equipment

> Eye patch
> Eye shield
> Silk tape

Psychosocial Considerations   The application of an eye patch or shield may cause anxiety in the child because he or she will not be able to see. This, coupled with the pain associated with the child's injury, may compound her or his distress.

Interventions should be aimed at keeping the child calm, as crying may cause an increase in intraocular pressure. Keep the child upright on the parent's lap. The young child may not want to keep the patch on his or her eye; soft elbow restraints may be necessary. Teach the child or parent how to care for the eye patch or shield at home.

Nursing responsibilities are described in Tables 11.2, 11.3, and 11.4.

Table 11.2.   Nursing Responsibilities

NURSING ACTIONS	RATIONALE
1. Explain to the child and the family the need for the eye patch or shield.	Enhances their understanding and cooperation.
2. Ensure that the eye has been properly treated.	
3. Apply the protective eye device. See Tables 11.3 and 11.4 for the procedures for an eye patch and an eye shield, respectively.	

Table 11.3.   Nursing Responsibilities for Applying an Eye Patch

NURSING ACTIONS	RATIONALE
1. To apply an eye patch,[4] place the child in a supine position; seek assistance to properly immobilize the child.	Prevents injury; the patch is applied firmly, to avoid further trauma to the cornea by blinking of the eyelid.[2]

Table 11.3.   *(cont.)*

NURSING ACTIONS	RATIONALE
2. Fold the first eye patch in half and place it over the closed eye.	
3. Place the second eye patch, fully opened, over the first patch.	
4. Apply tape to the child's cheek, then pull it upward over the patches, and anchor it onto the child's forehead.	
5. Patch the other eye in the same manner, if ordered by the physician.	
6. Document the treatment given, the presence of the patch, and how the child tolerated the procedure.	Communicates the nursing interventions and observations to other health-care professionals.

Table 11.4.   Nursing Responsibilities for Applying an Eye Shield

NURSING ACTIONS	RATIONALE
1. To apply an eye shield, allow the child to sit upright, either on the parent's lap or on the stretcher.	
2. Place the eye shield over the closed injured eye, making sure that it covers the orbit.	
3. Apply tape to the child's cheek, then pull it upward over the shield, and anchor it onto the child's forehead.	
4. Document the treatment given, the presence of the shield, and how the child tolerated the procedure.	Communicates the nursing interventions and observations to other health-care professionals.

EAR IRRIGATION

Indications   Ears are irrigated to remove cerumen or a foreign body.

Contraindications   Ruptured tympanic membrane; an unknown foreign body or one that may swell upon contact with water.

Complications   Possible trauma to the tympanic membrane or ear canal or obstruction of the ear canal, further inhibiting foreign-body removal. If the water temperature varies or the irrigation is rapid, the child could experience vertigo, nystagmus, or syncope.[1]

Equipment

> One 60-cc syringe
> Water Pik®
> Towels
> Basin
> One 18- or 20-gauge IV catheter sheath

Hydrogen peroxide
Warm water
Ear curette
Right angle hook
Alligator forceps
Suction device
Papoose board, if needed
Gloves

Psychosocial Considerations   Toddlers are very curious about their body openings and may insert objects into them. They consider any attempts by others to look into or touch their ears as intrusive, and they become very distressed, especially if the ear is already painful. If a Water Pik® is used, tell the child that the water will sound loud, but that he or she should not be frightened. Squirting some water on the child's hand before entering the ear canal may allay anxiety and gain trust. Encouraging the parent to comfort the child gives the parents a role in the procedure.

Nursing responsibilities are described in Table 11.5.

Table 11.5.   Nursing Responsibilities

NURSING ACTIONS	RATIONALE
1. Explain to the child and the family the need for ear irrigation.	Enhances their understanding and cooperation.
2. Place the child in a supine position, with towels placed under the neck and the head. If the child is uncooperative, additional restraint may be necessary (see Chapter 3).	Keeps child warm and dry.
3. Fill the basin with tepid water; for cerumen removal, add enough hydrogen peroxide to make a half-strength solution.	Facilitates removal of the foreign body or the cerumen.
4. Hold the basin below the child's ear. If an older child is cooperative, allow her or him to hold the basin.	Collects the solution and the wax or foreign body.
5. Fill the syringe, or turn on the Water Pik®. Place the catheter or the Water Pik® inside the external auditory canal, and direct the stream of water against the wall of the canal.[5]	
a. Gently pull the pinna downward and back for children less than 3 years old.[6]	Straightens ear canal.
b. Gently pull the pinna upward and back for children older than 3 years.	Straightens ear canal.
6. Stop the instillation of fluid if the child complains of pain or dizziness.[5] Irrigate for 10–15 minutes.[5]	Prevents complications.

Table 11.5.   (*cont.*)

NURSING ACTIONS	RATIONALE
7. Examine the solution for foreign body or for cerumen particles.	Determines the effectiveness of treatment.
8. Gently pat the child's head and neck dry; keep the child's head tilted.	Facilitates drainage of water from canal.
9. Examine the child's ear for visibility of the tympanic membrane, and notify physician if the foreign body or cerumen remains. Repeat the procedure, as indicated.	
10. Release the child from the securing device and praise the child for cooperating. Encourage the parent to comfort the child.	Gives the child a sense of control.
11. If the foreign body is still visualized in the ear, prepare for other options, as ordered by the physician:	
a. Removal by use of alligator forceps, low suction, or ear hook.	
b. Removal under general anesthesia if the child is struggling and the foreign body is still present.	
12. If cerumen is still present but softened, removal with an ear curette may be necessary.	
13. Document the effectiveness of the procedure and how the child tolerated the procedure.	Communicates the nursing interventions and observations to other health-care professionals.

ASSISTING WITH REMOVAL OF A FOREIGN BODY FROM THE NOSE

Indication   Foreign bodies are removed to prevent aspiration and local tissue necrosis.

Contraindications   Severe maxillofacial trauma, inability to visualize the foreign body, or an object that is deeply embedded, which requires removal under general anesthesia. The foreign body should never be pushed or irrigated into the nasopharynx, where it could be aspirated by the struggling child.[7]

Complications   Trauma to the nasal mucosa, causing epistaxis or swelling of tissue, which may further obstruct the nasal passages, aspiration of the foreign body; incomplete removal of the foreign body; rhinosinusitis.[7]

Equipment

   Light source (e.g., head lamp)
   Nasal speculum
   Nose drops (ephedrine, local anesthetic)

Alligator forceps / suction
Right angle hook
Papoose board (optional)
Gloves

Psychosocial Considerations   Foreign bodies of the nose are common in toddlers. The presence of a foreign body may not be suspected until the child has a purulent or malodorous nasal discharge. Talk calmly to the child during the procedure and explain what the child will feel. Securing the child in the papoose board may be necessary to avoid damaging the nasal mucosa while retrieving the foreign body. The parents can assist by distracting and comforting the child, if they are comfortable being present for this procedure.

Nursing responsibilities are described in Table 11.6.

PRESERVATION OF THE AVULSED TOOTH

Indications   Avulsed permanent teeth are preserved to enhance their viability for successful replantation. The best prognosis exists if therapy is instituted within $1/2$ hour of the avulsion.[8,9]

Table 11.6. Nursing Responsibilities

NURSING ACTIONS	RATIONALE
1. Explain to the child and the family the need for the procedure.	Enhances their understanding and cooperation.
2. Place the child in a supine position; if needed, restrain the child (see Chapter 3).	Facilitates completion of procedure and prevents further injury.
3. Instill a topical vasoconstrictor–anesthetic agent to shrink the swollen mucosa.[7] Consider a topical anesthetic if the procedure is prolonged or painful.	Promotes visualization of the foreign body and the ease of its removal.
4. The physician inserts the nasal speculum into the affected naris.	Enhances visualization of object.
5. Removal is accomplished with the use of low-level suction, a right angle hook, or alligator forceps. If the foreign body is not removed, or if the child is struggling, consider additional local anesthetic, or prepare the child for an examination under general anesthesia.	
6. Upon successful removal, release the child from the securing device and praise the child for cooperating.	Promotes a sense of mastery and control.
7. Document the object removed and how the child tolerated the procedure.	Communicate the nursing interventions and observations to other health-care professionals.

Contraindications   Replantation of avulsed primary teeth is generally not indicated because of the close proximity of the permanent teeth to the socket.[8]

Complications   Ingestion or aspiration of the avulsed tooth; damage to periodontal ligaments of the root during replacement of the tooth into the socket.[8]

Psychosocial Considerations   Dental trauma frequently occurs in the younger child, due to his or her developing mobility and sense of exploration. Although replantation of the primary tooth is generally not indicated, the parent should be reassured that this injury rarely results in problems with permanent dentition.

It is helpful to reassure the older child, in whom body image is paramount, that prompt and appropriate treatment should result in saving the tooth. Instruct children who participate in contact sports about the use of properly fitting mouthguards, to reduce the incidence of further dental injuries.

Nursing responsibilities are described in Table 11.7.

Table 11.7.   Nursing Responsibilities

NURSING ACTIONS	RATIONALE
1. Explain to the child and the family how the tooth is preserved.	Enhances their understanding and cooperation.
2. Gently rinse the tooth with tap water; do not scrub the tooth or remove attached tissue.[8]	Scrubbing the tooth may cause further damage.
3. Determine the presence of other oral injuries that would prevent replantation. Reimplant the tooth by holding the crown, concave side toward the back and gently pushing it into socket.	Grasping the tooth by the crown may prevent further damage to the periodontal ligaments.
4. If unable to reimplant the tooth, have the child hold the tooth under the tongue.[8] Do not attempt this step if the child is either too young to understand not to swallow the tooth or is in an altered state of consciousness.	Decreases risk of ingestion or aspiration of the tooth.
5. If unable to accomplish Steps 3 and 4, place the tooth in milk,[8] label the cup with the child's name and the time this measure was instituted.	Milk or saliva is the best medium to maintain the periodontal ligament and vitality.[8]
6. Consult a dentist or oral maxillofacial surgeon for further treatment.	Prompt treatment may prevent the loss of permanent teeth.
7. Document the child's condition, the time of injury, and the specific methods initiated for tooth preservation.	Communicates the nursing interventions and observations to other health-care professionals.

REFERENCES

1. Hughes W, Buescher E. Pediatric procedures. 2nd ed. Philadelphia: W.B. Saunders, 1980;192,202.
2. Goodale LS. Ophthalmic emergencies. In: Kelley S, ed. Pediatric emergency nursing. Norwalk, CT: Appleton-Lange, 1988; 245–246,249.
3. Diamond GR. Ophthalmic emergencies. In: Fleischer G, Ludwig S, eds. Textbook of pediatric emergency medicine. 2nd ed. Baltimore: Williams & Wilkins, 1988;997.
4. Thompson SW. Emergency care of children. Boston: Jones & Bartlett, 1990;188.
5. Servonsky J, Opas SR. Nursing management of children. Boston: Jones & Bartlett, 1987;1253.
6. Dutton L. Administering medications. In: Nursing '85 books: Nursing photo series. Nursing pediatric patients. Springhouse, PA: Springhouse Corp., 1985;66.
7. Ruddy RM. Procedures. In: Fleisher G, Ludwig S, eds. Textbook of pediatric emergency medicine. 2nd ed. Baltimore: Williams & Wilkins, 1988;1287.
8. Nelson LP, Neff JH. Dental emergencies. In: Fleisher G, Ludwig S, eds. Textbook of pediatric emergency medicine. 2nd ed. Baltimore: Williams & Wilkins, 1988;1104.
9. Broring C. Dental injuries. In: Mayer T, ed. Emergency management of pediatric trauma. Philadelphia: W.B. Saunders, 1985;323.

12

Medication Administration

Kathleen O'Connor

OVERVIEW OF PEDIATRIC MEDICATION ADMINISTRATION

Administering medications to children poses a unique challenge for the emergency nurse. The nurse must be aware of the child's developmental age and the most effective methods for approaching each age group when administering medications. Children may be sensitive to medications and may have severe reactions to some of them. This sensitivity and reactivity may be due to children's higher metabolic rates, which affect the absorption, metabolism, and excretion of the medication.

Parents can serve as allies when administering medications. In some cases, it is less traumatic for the child to have the parent administer the medication, with the nurse supervising the process. Alternatively, parents may be able to give insights that help the nurse administer the medication without a struggle.

Parents should be kept informed of the medications their child is receiving. Taking a few minutes to answer their questions will allay their fears and build a trusting rapport with the emergency nurse. Also, in some situations, parents may need to practice medication administration before leaving the emergency department (ED).

Five essential steps must *always* be followed when administering medications to any patient. Ascertain the following:

1. *Correct patient*   Check the child's name on the ED identification band.
2. *Correct medication*   Check the physician's order for the correct name of the medication, and know the indication for its prescribed use. Carefully inspect the label of the medication to be administered so that it corresponds to the physician's order.
3. *Correct dose*   Check the medication references to ensure that the dose is within the safe range for the child's weight.
4. *Correct time*   Check the medication reference and the physician's order to make sure that the timing of administration is correct.
5. *Correct route*   Check the references and the physician's order to ensure that the prescribed intended route is acceptable.

ADMINISTRATION OF OPHTHALMIC MEDICATIONS

Indications   Ophthalmic medications are administered to treat infection, moisten the eyes, or provide anesthesia before examination or irrigation of the eyes.

Contraindications   Known sensitivity to medication; not recommended if the eyelids cannot be opened or if penetrating eye trauma is present.

Complications   Adverse reaction to medication.

Equipment

> Medication—the label should read, "For ophthalmic use"
> Clean cotton balls
> Sterile normal saline solution (NSS)

Psychosocial Considerations   Children need reassurance that changes in their vision are temporary; it is often helpful to have them close their eyes and relax by telling a story or encouraging progressive relaxation.

Teach the parents how to administer eye medications at home if indicated.

Nursing responsibilities are described in Table 12.1.

ADMINISTRATION OF OTIC MEDICATIONS

Indications   Ear drops are administered for pain relief, treatment of an external ear infection, or cerumen removal.

Contraindications   Known sensitivity to medication; not recommended if there is a possibility of a basilar skull fracture; in addition, many types of ear drops should not be administered if the ear drum is perforated.[1]

Complications   The presence of a cerebrospinal fluid (CSF) leak into the ear increases the risk of meningitis; ear drops should not be given when such a communication with the central nervous system (CNS) exists.[1] Adverse reaction to the medication.

Equipment

> Medication
> Clean cotton ball
> NSS
> Gloves

Psychosocial Considerations   Young children who require ear drops often have an ear infection or cerumen buildup, either of which can be painful. Manipulating the ear under these circumstances can increase the child's discomfort. Also, being held securely for the procedure creates additional frustration in the young child.

The parents can help by holding the child or talking to her or him during the procedure. Providing distraction helps to keep the child still so that the medication can take effect.

Table 12.1. Nursing Responsibilities

NURSING ACTIONS	RATIONALE
1. Check the medication order for the dosage, amount, time, and route. Check the child's ED identification band; assess for any medication allergies.	Ensures proper medication administration to the correct child.
2. Hold the bottle of medication up to the light (if the medication bottle is translucent). Check the expiration date.	Allows for visualization of sediment or a change in color. Do not use the medication if either is present.
3. Warm the solution to body temperature between your hands for a few minutes.	All ophthalmic medication should be administered at body temperature.
4. Wash your hands; don gloves, if needed.	Minimizes the spread of infection.
5. Explain to the child and the family the need for the ophthalmic medication. Explain that the ointment or drops may temporarily blur the child's vision.	Enhances their understanding and cooperation.
6. Place the child in a supine position with the head tilted back and slightly turned toward the affected eye.[2] Use a pillow or shoulder roll. Place infants and young children supine on the parent's lap with their neck slightly extended. The struggling child may need to be secured in this position by a parent or by another health professional.	Helps dispense the ophthalmic medication into the eye, away from the lacrimal duct.[3]
7. Wipe the child's eyelid with a cotton ball moistened with NSS, from the inner canthus outward in one stroke. Use a separate cotton ball for each stroke. Continue until any crusted material is removed.	Cleanses lashes and lids. Removes debris and prevents the spread of infection.
8. Wipe the opposite eyelid in the same manner with another moistened cotton ball.	
9. Rest hand that will administer the medication on the child's forehead or cheek.	
10. With the opposite hand, place your thumb on the child's cheekbone and gently pull down the lower eyelid or open the eye with your second and third fingers.	Exposes the conjunctival sac for administration of the medication.[3]

Table 12.1. *(cont.)*

NURSING ACTIONS	RATIONALE
11. Ask the child to look up and to the opposite side, if possible.	Avoids placing medication directly onto the cornea.
12. Administer the medication.	
a. *Drops:* Instill the prescribed number of drops into the lower outer part of the conjunctival sac, being careful not to touch the eye or lashes with the bottle (see Figure 12.1).	Prevents contamination of the dropper.

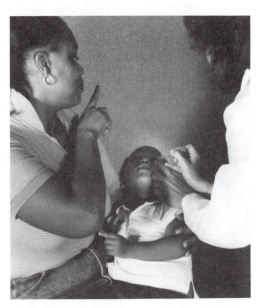

Figure 12.1. Positioning a child for administration of eye drops. The mother is instructing the child to look upward. If necessary, her right hand can be used to secure the child's left arm.

b. *Ointment:* Place a line of ointment in the inner margin of the lower lid, starting at the inner canthus and moving toward the outer canthus.[4] Eye ointments are intended for single patient use only.	Avoids placement on the cornea.
13. After instilling the medication ask the child to close his or her eyes gently, or do it for the child, for approximately 2 minutes.[4] Hold a cotton ball gently over the inner canthus.	Makes medication more effective by spreading medicine around eye; helps prevent the solution from entering the lacrimal duct.
14. Repeat the foregoing procedure if	

Table 12.1.   (*cont.*)

NURSING ACTIONS	RATIONALE
medication also is indicated for the opposite eye.	
15. Praise the child for cooperating; wash your hands.	
16. Document the type of eye medication administered, the dosage, the time of administration, the eye that was treated, and how the child tolerated the procedure.	Communicates the nursing interventions and observations to health-care professionals.

Teach the parent how to administer nasal medications at home, if indicated.

Nursing responsibilities are described in Table 12.2.

Table 12.2.   Nursing Responsibilities

NURSING ACTIONS	RATIONALE
1. Check the medication order for dosage, amount, time, and route. Check the child's ED identification band; assess for medication allergies.	Ensures proper medication administration to the correct child.
2. Warm the solution to body temperature by holding the bottle between your hands for a few minutes.[5]	Administration of cold solution in the ears may cause pain or vertigo.
3. Wash your hands; don gloves, if needed.	Minimizes spread of infection.
4. Explain to the child and the family the need for the ear drops.	Enhances their understanding and cooperation.
5. Turn the child's head so that the affected side is up. Additional assistance may be necessary to secure a young child.	Exposes the affected ear, to administer the medication.
6. Cleanse the ear with a clean cotton ball moistened with NSS.	
7. For children less than 3 years old, gently pull the pinna *downward* and back.[6]	Straightens ear canal.
For children older than 3 years, gently pull the pinna *upward* and back.	Straightens the ear canal.
8. Instill the prescribed number of drops into the external canal, being careful not to touch the ear with the dropper.	Prevents contamination of the dropper.
9. Gently massage the area immediately anterior to the ear, to facilitate the entry of drops into ear.[6]	Permits medication to run down ear canal easily.

Table 12.2. (*cont.*)

NURSING ACTIONS	RATIONALE
10. Keep the child in this position for approximately 10 minutes. If unable to keep the child in this position, insert a medication-soaked cotton ball in the external ear canal.	Increases absorption of the medication.
11. Wash your hands; praise the child for cooperating.	
12. Document the medication, the dosage, the time of administration, the ear that was treated, and how the child tolerated the procedure.	Communicates the nursing interventions and observations to health-care professionals.

ADMINISTRATION OF NASAL MEDICATIONS

Indications   Nasal medications are administered to decrease nasal congestion and to anesthetize the nare for procedures.

Contraindications   Known sensitivity to medication; maxillofacial trauma.

Complications   Meningitis when basilar skull fracture and CSF rhinorrhea are present. Adverse reaction to the medication.

Equipment

> Medication bottle with dropper or spray
> Tissues
> Gloves

Psychosocial Considerations   Young children may perceive this procedure as intrusive, because it involves manipulation of a body opening. Children need to know that they should extend their necks to avoid feeling the medicine trickling down their throat.[5]

Parents can participate by distracting and comforting the child. Teach the parent how to administer nasal medications at home, if indicated.

Nursing responsibilities are described in Table 12.3.

Table 12.3. Nursing Responsibilities

NURSING ACTIONS	RATIONALE
1. Check the medication order for the dosage, amount, time, and route. Check the child's ED identification band; assess for any medication allergies.	Ensures proper medication administration to the correct child.
2. Hold the bottle of medication up to the light (if the bottle is translucent). Check the expiration date.	Allows for visualization of sediment or a change in color. Do not use the medication if either is present.

Table 12.3. (*cont.*)

NURSING ACTIONS	RATIONALE
3. Warm the solution to body temperature between your hands for a few minutes.	Nasal medication should be administered at body temperature.
4. Wash your hands; don gloves if needed.	Minimizes the spread of infection.
5. Explain to the child and the family the need for the nasal medication.	Enhances their understanding and cooperation.
6. Position the child for the procedure (see Figure 12.2).	Allows for proper absorption of the medication.

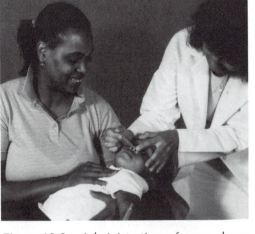

Figure 12.2. Administration of nose drops to a young child. Note how the mother secures the child by allowing his right arm to encircle her waist, thus reducing movement. With her right hand, she is able to control the child's free arm. To provide him with some control, the child is allowed to hold onto a clean dropper.

a. *Infants and younger children:* Position them supine across the parent's arm, with their head tilted back; the parent can hold the child's arms with the free hand.	
b. *Older children:* Have the child lie supine with the head tilted back; a pillow or towel roll may be placed under the shoulders.[6]	
7. Suction the nares with a bulb syringe three to four times,[7] if needed.	Clears the nasal passages of any secretions.
8. Prepare the prescribed amount of medication in the dropper; insert	Inserting the tip of dropper or sprayer allows for drop counting and

Table 12.3. *(cont.)*

NURSING ACTIONS	RATIONALE
the tip of the dropper or sprayer only slightly into the nares. Instill the ordered amount of drops into the upper part of nostril.	minimizes any trauma to the nares.
9. Keep the child in the same position for approximately 1 minute. Observe for any signs of aspiration; if the child coughs, hold him or her upright. Instruct the child not to blow her or his nose. Tell an older child to breathe through his or her mouth.[6]	Allows for absorption of medication.
10. Rinse the dropper with warm water.	
11. Praise the child for cooperating; wash your hands.	
12. Document the type of nasal medication administered, the time of administration, the naris that was treated, and how the child tolerated the procedure.	Communicates the nursing interventions and observations to health-care professionals.

ADMINISTRATION OF ORAL MEDICATIONS

Indications   Oral administration of medications is used in the conscious, awake child. The child's cooperation must be gained in order for the medication to be swallowed and retained. Medications for oral use are supplied in the forms of tablets, capsules, caplets, or liquids.

Contraindications   Known sensitivity to the medication; unconsciousness; airway obstruction, respiratory distress, nothing by mouth (NPO) status, intubated children. The child must have a gag reflex and the ability to swallow.

Complications   Vomiting and aspiration. Adverse reaction to the medication.

Equipment

> Medication for administration
> Syringe/dropper
> Medicine cup
> Mortar and pestle (for crushing tablets)
> Gloves

Psychosocial Considerations   The method of administering oral medications is based on the child's developmental stage and on insights provided by the parents. Infants require liquid medications. Toddlers and preschoolers may prefer a chewable tablet or may take a tablet that is crushed and sprinkled over a small amount of food, such as applesauce. Tell the child that the medication is mixed with the food because she or he may be able to taste it.

Allow the child a choice whenever possible, such as the type of food in which to mix the medication, the kind of container in which to put it, or what to drink after taking the medication. Do not ask the child whether he or she wants to take the medicine; the child will invariably say "no," and a struggle will ensue. The school-age child can either take liquid or chewable medications or may be able to swallow a capsule or tablet.[6] Adolescents can usually take any form of oral medication.

Nursing responsibilities are described in Tables 12.4 through 12.9.

Table 12.4. Nursing Responsibilities

NURSING ACTIONS	RATIONALE
1. Check the medication order for the dosage, amount, time, and route. Check the child's ED identification band; assess for any medication allergies.	Ensures proper medication administration to the correct child.
2. Check the expiration date.	
3. Wash your hands; don gloves, if needed.	Minimizes the spread of infection.
4. Prepare a proper dose of the medication, either in a syringe without a needle, in a dropper, or in a medication cup.	Ensures accuracy of dosage.
5. Explain to the child and the family the need for the medication.	Enhances their understanding and cooperation.
6. Have the parent hold the child on his or her lap in an upright position, with the head slightly tilted back. If the child is not cooperative, secure her or him by having the parent hug the child.	Promotes ease of administration and security for the child. Decreases the chance of aspiration.
7. Administer the medication, as indicated in Tables 12.5 through 12.9.	
8. Praise the child for cooperating.	Gives the child a sense of mastery.
9. Wash your hands.	
10. If the child vomits immediately after administration, notify the physician, as the dose may need to be repeated.	
11. Document the medication dosage, the time of administration, and how the child tolerated the procedure.	Communicates the nursing interventions and observations to health-care professionals.

Table 12.5. Syringe or Dropper Method

NURSING ACTIONS	RATIONALE
1. Administer liquid medication no more than ½ cc at a time, between the child's cheek and gum.	Facilitates swallowing and prevents aspiration.
2. Wait until the child swallows that amount before administering more of the medication (see Figure 12.3).	

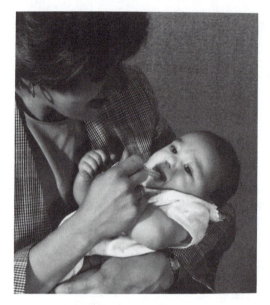

Figure 12.3.   Administration of an oral medication to an infant, using the syringe method. Note how the mother secures the infant's left hand to prevent movement and positions the baby upright to facilitate swallowing.

Table 12.6. Nipple Method

NURSING ACTIONS	RATIONALE
1. Place the medication in a nipple.	Takes advantage of the infant's sucking ability.
2. Do not mix the medication with formula.	The infant may not drink formula afterward, because it tastes different; promotes distrust.
3. Pour about 5 cc of sterile water into the nipple after the infant has sucked the medication.	Clears the nipple of all medications.

Table 12.7.   Chewable Tablet

NURSING ACTIONS	RATIONALE
Determine which fluids are compatible with the medication; give the child a choice as to what she or he wants to drink with the medication.	

Table 12.8.   Crushable Tablet/Caplet

NURSING ACTIONS	RATIONALE
1. Do not crush enteric-coated tablets.	The medication will not be absorbed properly. The tablets are coated so that they are digested in the small intestine.
2. Place the tablet in a mortar and crush the pill with the pestle.	Enables better dilution.
3. In a small measuring cup, mix the crushed tablet and the premeasured amount of fluid, which should be minimal.	
4. Use sterile water, Kool-Aid™, apple juice, or any fluid that is compatible with the medication. Avoid using formula or milk as the base for mixing the medication.	The child will be able to taste the medication and may no longer accept formula or milk.

Table 12.9.   Capsules

NURSING ACTIONS	RATIONALE
May be diluted and administered like tablets, but caution should be taken with "time released" capsules; check with the pharmacist before diluting such capsules.	Absorption of medication can be affected.

ADMINISTRATION OF RECTAL MEDICATION

Indications   Medications are administered rectally in the child who is vomiting or is NPO, is in respiratory distress, or has a decreased level of consciousness. Rectal administration eliminates the risk of aspiration and does not irritate the stomach.

Contraindications   Known sensitivity to the medication; rectal bleeding, rectal prolapse, increased intracranial pressure, coagulopathy, neutropenia, an acute surgical abdomen, acute ulcerative colitis, or recent rectal surgery.[1]

Complications   Perforation or injury to the rectum, sepsis, bleeding; adverse reaction to the medication.

Equipment

Gloves
Water-soluble lubricant
Washcloth
Medication (suppository)

Psychosocial Considerations   Children and adolescents are very modest about their bodies. Reassure the child that he or she will feel "pressure" but will not defecate; know which word the child uses for defecation. Ask the parents to help by distracting the child and practicing deep breathing techniques.

Nursing responsibilities are described in Table 12.10.

Table 12.10.   Nursing Responsibilities

NURSING ACTIONS	RATIONALE
1. Check the medication order for the dosage, amount, time, and route; check the child's ED identification band; assess for any medication allergies.	Ensures proper administration of the medication to the correct child.
2. Check the expiration date.	
3. Explain to the child and the family the need for the rectal medication.	Enhances their understanding and cooperation.
4. Pull the curtains, or close the door.	Provides privacy.
5. Wash your hands; don gloves.	Prevents transmission of infection.
6. Position the child on her or his left side, with the right leg drawn up, or on the back, with legs flexed (infants and toddlers).	Allows for entrance of medication into the rectum.
7. Lubricate the tapered tip end of the suppository.	Allows for ease of insertion.
8. Gently separate the buttocks and expose the anus.	
9. Ask the child to breathe deeply through the mouth if the child can understand this instruction. Hold the suppository in your dominant hand; insert the tapered end past the anal sphincter, along the rectal wall. Ensure that the suppository is not inserted into fecal material.	Distraction promotes relaxation of the anal sphincter; allows for adequate absorption of medication.
10. Hold the buttocks together for 1–2 minutes after insertion.[4]	Ensures that the suppository will not be expelled.
11. Clean the excess lubricant from the child's anus.	Promotes comfort.
12. Praise the child for cooperating.	Provides a sense of mastery.

Table 12.10.   (*cont.*)

NURSING ACTIONS	RATIONALE
13. Remove the gloves, and wash your hands.	Minimizes the spread of infection.
14. Document the medication dosage, the time of administration, and how the child tolerated the procedure.	Communicates the nursing interventions and observations to health-care professionals.

ADMINISTRATION OF AN ENEMA

Indications   Enemas are indicated to cleanse the bowel and to treat constipation.

Contraindications   Enemas are not administered in conjunction with rectal bleeding or rectal prolapse.[1]

Complications   Bowel perforation or injury, water intoxication, or transient bacteremia.[8]

Equipment

> Bedpan/diaper/potty chair
> Gloves
> Washcloth
> Enema solution to be administered

Psychosocial Considerations   Children and adolescents are very modest about their bodies, especially their private areas. Preschoolers pride themselves on using a potty chair or toilet and can become distressed if they soil themselves. School-age children and adolescents may also fear not being able to "hold" an enema or not getting to the toilet in time. Adolescents who ingest balloons or condoms filled with illegal drugs will need to use a bedpan, usually in the presence of narcotics officers, who will then retrieve the evidence.

Know which word the young child uses for defecation so that the child understands what will happen. The child may feel out of control with the expulsion of an enema; praise the child for his or her efforts and offer reassurance. Ask the parents to help by distracting the child. Cleaning the child shortly after the enema takes effect will help the child to feel comfortable.

Nursing responsibilities are described in Table 12.11.

Table 12.11.   Nursing Responsibilities

NURSING ACTIONS	RATIONALE
1. Check the medication order for the dosage, amount, time, and route. Check the child's ED identification band; assess for any medication allergies.	Ensures proper administration of the medication to the correct child.

Table 12.11.   *(cont.)*

NURSING ACTIONS	RATIONALE
2. Warm the enema in a basin of tepid water for about 20 minutes.	Warms to body temperature.
3. Explain to the child and the family the need for the enema.	Promotes their understanding and cooperation.
4. Wash your hands; don gloves.	Ensures clean technique.
5. Pull the curtain, or close the door.	Promotes privacy.
6. Place a bed pad under the child's buttocks, and place the child in one of the following positions:[8]	Exposes the anal area for insertion.
a. on left side with right leg flexed about 45 degrees (Sims position).	Allows for entrance of the enema into the colon.
b. on abdomen with knees drawn up (knee–chest)	
c. on left side in the lateral decubitus position, with knees drawn up to chest	
d. placed on back, with legs flexed (infant or toddler).	
7. Remove the plastic tip from the enema bottle or tubing.	
8. Ask the child to take a few deep breaths; gently insert the bottle tip or tubing into the rectum. See Table 12.12 to determine the appropriate length for the tube insertion.	Helps the child to relax, for ease of administration.
9. Slowly administer the fluid. If the child shows symptoms of distress, immediately stop the flow of the solution.[8]	
10. Remove the bottle tip or tubing, and hold the buttocks together for a few minutes, until the child's urge to defecate becomes strong.[7]	Ensures action of enema.
11. Assist the child to the toilet, potty chair, or bedpan, or place a diaper on the infant.	Allows for measurement of the eliminated stool.
12. Remove the gloves, and wash your hands.	Minimizes the spread of infection.
13. Praise the child for cooperating.	Instills a sense of mastery and control.
14. Document how the child tolerated the procedure, the time of administration, the type and amount of enema given, and a description of the	Communicates the nursing intervention and observations to health-care professionals.

Table 12.11.   *(cont.)*

NURSING ACTIONS	RATIONALE
amount, appearance, and odor of the stool. Document the presence of any evidence and who collected the evidence (narcotics officer).	

Table 12.12.   Guidelines for Enema Tube Length, Size, and Fluid Amount[2]

AGES	TUBE LENGTH	FLUID AMOUNT
Infants up to 2 years	1–1$^1/_2$"	250 cc or less
Children 2–6 years	1$^1/_2$–2"	500 cc or less
Children 6–12 years	2–3"	500–1000 cc
Adolescents	3–4"	750–1000 cc

ADMINISTRATION OF TOPICAL MEDICATION

Indications   Topical medications are used to anesthetize the skin for suturing, relieve pruritis, prevent infection, and reduce inflammation.

Contraindications   Known sensitivity to medication.

Complications   Toxic absorption of medication if applied too liberally or indiscriminately; local irritation; adverse reaction to the medication.

Equipment

> Medication
> Gloves
> Cotton-tipped applicators
> Sterile gauze pads

Psychosocial Considerations   Infants and toddlers may try to eat or lick the medication if it is on a hand or finger that they normally suck for comfort. In this case, a pacifier may be substituted; if appropriate, cover the areas where the medication was applied.
   Nursing responsibilities are described in Table 12.13.

ADMINISTRATION OF SUBCUTANEOUS MEDICATIONS

Indications   The subcutaneous route is used to administer small amounts of medication into the subcutaneous tissues. The usual dose is 0.5–1.0 cc.[3]

Contraindications   Known sensitivity to medication; medications in heavy

Table 12.13. Nursing Responsibilities

NURSING ACTIONS	RATIONALE
1. Check the medication order for the dosage, amount, time, and route. Check the child's ED identification band; assess for medication allergies.	Ensures proper administration of the medication to the correct child.
2. Wash your hands; don gloves, if needed.	Minimizes the spread of infection.
3. Explain to the child and the family the need for the medication.	Enhances their understanding and cooperation.
4. Wash the area with mild soap and warm water, if indicated.	
5. Open the medication container, or remove the lid. Place the lid upright, or place it on a gauze pad.	Prevents contamination of the lid.
6. Apply the medication, as ordered, to the affected area, using either of two methods: (1) with a single cotton-tipped applicator, wipe from the affected area outward, using one applicator for each stroke; (2) with a glove, place medication on the gloved fingers, and use short strokes to gently apply the medication to the affected area.	Prevents the spread of infection.
7. Apply a dressing, if ordered (see Chapter 10).	Allows for absorption of medication.
8. Praise the child for cooperating; wash your hands.	
9. Document how the child tolerated the procedure, the time of administration, and the type of medication administered and the area to which the medication was applied.	Communicates the nursing interventions and observations to health-care professionals.

suspensions or irritant medications;[8] solutions greater than 1.5 cc. If the rate of absorption is a concern, do not use this route.

Complications   Tissue damage; adverse reaction to the medication.

Equipment

>   2 × 2 gauze pad
>   Alcohol wipes
>   Band-Aid™
>   25–26 gauge needle, size 3/8″ for infant or thin child, 5/8″ for larger child[3]
>   3 cc syringe or smaller
>   Gloves

Psychosocial Considerations   Children fear injections because they do not like the discomfort of the injection or of being secured. Explain to the child what he or she will feel (coolness, a pinch, a burning feeling). Encourage the older child to concentrate on her or his breathing, to count to 10, or use some other distraction technique. Praise the child for being cooperative, and encourage the parents to comfort their child afterward. Older children and adolescents can administer their own insulin, under the observation of the emergency nurse.

Nursing responsibilities are described in Table 12.14.

Table 12.14. Nursing Responsibilities

NURSING ACTIONS	RATIONALE
1. Check the medication order for the dosage, amount, time, and route. Check the child's ED identification band; assess for medication allergies.	Ensures proper administration of medication to the correct patient.
2. Explain to the child and the family the need for the medication.	Enhances their understanding and cooperation.
3. Wash your hands; don gloves.	Minimizes the spread of infection.
4. Select the site for subcutaneous injection: upper arm, anterior thigh, anterior abdominal wall, or inter- or subscapular areas.[3] Clean the site with an alcohol wipe.	
5. Obtain additional assistance from other health-care professionals, if needed.	
6. Gently grasp the child's skin between your thumb and forefinger.	Isolates the subcutaneous layer.[1]
7. Insert the needle at a 90-degree angle; withdraw the plunger slightly, to observe for any blood in the syringe. If blood is observed, a blood vessel has been entered. Remove the syringe immediately, and discard it. Prepare new medication with a new needle and syringe, and repeat the foregoing steps, as needed.	
8. Inject the medication.	
9. Withdraw the syringe and needle quickly, at the same angle in which it was inserted.	
10. Apply slight pressure to the site with a sterile 2 × 2 gauze pad; gently massage the site, if indicated. Apply a Band-Aid™.	Prevents medication leak from the site; increases circulation and enhances absorption.
11. Comfort and praise the child; wash your hands.	Provides a sense of mastery.
12. Document the medication and the dosage administered, the site for administration, the time it was admin-	Communicates the nursing interventions and observations to health-care professionals.

Table 12.14. *(cont.)*

NURSING ACTIONS	RATIONALE
istered, how the child tolerated the procedure, and any changes in the child's condition following the medication administration.	

ADMINISTRATION OF INTRADERMAL INJECTIONS

Indications The intradermal route is used for immunization, desensitization, or diagnostic skin tests.[8]

Contraindications Known sensitivity to the medication or test. Intradermal injections are not administered in areas that are burned, injured, or neurovascularly impaired. Volumes greater than 0.1 cc should not be administered by this route.[3]

Complications Allergic reaction to antigens; inadvertent injection into the subcutaneous tissue.[8]

Equipment

>   Tuberculin
>   Syringe (tb)
>   25-gauge ⁵/₈″ needle[3]
>   Alcohol wipes
>   2 × 2 gauze pads
>   Band-Aid™
>   Gloves

Psychosocial Considerations Intradermal skin testing is uncomfortable for the child. Explain to the child what he or she will feel (coolness, a pinch). Encourage the child to participate, if she or he shows an interest, by holding the Band-Aid™. Comfort the child during and after the injection.

   Nursing responsibilities are described in Table 12.15.

Table 12.15. Nursing Responsibilities

NURSING ACTIONS	RATIONALE
1. Check the medication order for the test or medication to be administered. Ensure the correct time, dosage and route. Check the child's ED identification band, and assess for any medication allergies.	Ensures proper administration of the test/medication to the correct child.
2. Wash your hands.	Prevents spread of infection.
3. Explain to the child and the family the need for the injection.	Enhances their understanding and cooperation.
4. Determine the site for intradermal injection; selected sites are the anterior aspect of the forearm, the intrascapular area, the anterior ab-	Ensures proper injection site.

Table 12.15.   (*cont.*)

NURSING ACTIONS	RATIONALE
dominal wall, and the inner aspect of the thigh.[8]	
5. Have the parent hold a younger child on her or his lap; have the older child sit upright. An assistant may be needed to help secure the child.	Prevents injury to the child.
6. Clean the selected site with an alcohol wipe.	Prevents contamination of the site.
7. Gently pull the skin taut with your hand. Position the needle, bevel up, against the skin. Enter the skin almost parallel with the skin surface, until the bevel disappears from view.[8]	
8. Slowly inject the solution to produce a bleb. If a bleb is not produced, the injection was probably delivered to the subcutaneous tissue and must be repeated at a new site.	Ensures proper placement of the solution.
9. Remove the needle, and apply pressure gently with a gauze sponge.	Promotes comfort.
10. Praise the child for cooperating; wash your hands.	Gives the child a sense of mastery.
11. Document the time, site, and test administered, as well as the child's response to the procedure. If a test was administered, ensure that the parents know when to return to have the test read.	Communicates the nursing interventions and observations to health-care professionals.

ADMINISTRATION OF INTRAMUSCULAR MEDICATIONS

Indications   A means to achieve relatively rapid medication effects when oral or IV routes are not indicated. The intramuscular route allows for the administration of medication to a child who is unconscious, unable to swallow, or fluid restricted. Aqueous suspensions, solutions in oil, or medications that do not come in oral form can be administered by this route.

Contraindications   Known sensitivity to the medication. Intramuscular (IM) injections are not given to children with severe burns, due to erratic absorption; nor are they administered in neurovascularly compromised extremities.

Complications   Damage to blood vessels, causing bleeding or improper absorption of the medication; nerve damage, causing pain or paralysis; and tissue, bone and muscle damage.[5] Adverse reaction to the medication.

Equipment

Alcohol wipes

Povidone–iodine wipes (for immunosuppressed children)

2 × 2 gauze pad

Band-Aid™

Appropriate needle and syringe size—for less than 1 cc of medication, use a tuberculin syringe

Gloves

Psychosocial Considerations   Younger children perceive injections as intrusive. Apply a Band-Aid™ to calm the child.

Infants have pain with injections, and by late infancy or early toddlerhood will associate the sight of a needle with pain. Young children also may associate receiving an injection with punishment. The word "shot" should be avoided, as this gives the impression of being shot with a gun; the words "injection" or "pinch" are less threatening. Older children may need to know that it is permissible to cry after an injection because they want to be "brave" and do not want anyone to know that it hurts. The child may not want to watch the injection procedure; ask the parent or your assistant to turn the child's head away from the injection site. Prepare the child for what she or he will feel (cool, pinch, burn). Let the child hold the Band-Aid™, if he or she wants to participate.

Parents may choose to leave during an injection. The parent may threaten or scold the child for not keeping still or cooperating; explain to the family that it is difficult for the child to keep still and that this is normal behavior. Children may try to stall the procedure; give the child a specified amount of time ("I'll count to 3, and then I'll give the injection") to help the child face the inevitable. Always praise and reward the child after the injection.

Nursing responsibilities are described in Table 12.16.

Table 12.16. Nursing Responsibilities

NURSING ACTIONS	RATIONALE
1. Check the medication order for the dosage, amount, time, and route. Check the child's ED identification band; assess for any medication allergies.	Ensures proper administration of the medication to the correct child.
2. Prepare the medication into syringe; change the needle to one appropriate for the selected injection site. Consider the child's muscle mass, size, nutritional status, viscosity of the medication, and amount of medication to be administered when selecting the needle size and injection site.	Prevents contamination of the injection site.

Table 12.16. (cont.)

NURSING ACTIONS	RATIONALE
a. Vastus lateralis—use 22- to 25-gauge ⁵/₈–1″ needle size.[5]	Preferred site for all ages; has a larger muscle mass, can tolerate greater amounts of fluid, and there are few major nerves or vessels in the area.[5]
b. Ventrogluteal and dorsogluteal—use 20- to 25-gauge 1–1¹/₂″.[5]	Only used in children over age 3 years and who have been walking for more than a year. The ventrogluteal muscle is large and has few nerves and blood vessels.[5]
c. Deltoid—use 22- to 25-gauge ¹/₂–1″.[5]	Faster absorption rates than gluteal sites. Limited amounts of medication are administered, due to smaller muscle mass.[5]
3. Prepare the child for injection.	
a. *Infants*—Avoid giving the infant a bottle during injections.	Reduces the risk of aspiration.
b. *Toddlers/preschoolers*—Distract the child from seeing the needle. Avoid using terms that suggest harm (e.g., *shot, stick*). Allow minimal time lapse between the explanation and the injection. Allow the child to select the injection site, if possible.	The child's concept of time is not well developed at this age.
c. *School-age children*—Briefly describe what you will do. "The injection will hurt but the pain will go away." Allow the child to select the injection site, if possible. Tell the child that it is okay to cry.	Able to understand cause and effect.
d. *Adolescents*—Privacy is very important. Be honest with them. Let them know that it is okay to cry. Allow them to select the injection site, if possible.	Strives for independence yet still has dependency needs; may be frightened.
4. Wash your hands; don gloves.	Minimizes the spread of infection.
5. Summon extra assistance, if needed, to help secure the child.	Avoids prolonging the injection.
6. Cleanse the injection site in a brisk circular motion with an alcohol wipe and let the area dry. For the immunosuppressed child, cleanse the site with povidone–iodine, wipe with alcohol, and let it dry.	Decreases skin microbes.
7. Ask the parent to comfort the child and provide distraction; the parent may want to hold the child's hands	

Table 12.16.   *(cont.)*

NURSING ACTIONS	RATIONALE

or arms while comforting the child
(see Figure 12.4).

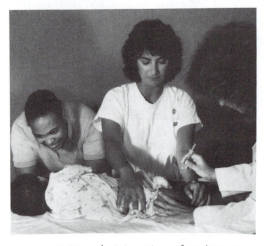

Figure 12.4.   Administration of an intramuscular medication. The mother distracts the child while one nurse secures the leg. In an older child, more than one nurse may be needed to assure proper immobilization for medication administration.

8. Encourage the awake and cooperative child to relax the muscle by wiggling her or his toes or fingers, focusing on another object, or counting.

    Makes the injection less painful.

9. Stretch the skin taut at the insertion site with the nondominant hand.

    Displaces the subcutaneous tissue for correct needle placement in the muscle.

10. Hold the syringe at the lower end. Insert the needle quickly at a 45–90-degree angle, depending on the selected site. Withdraw the plunger slightly, and observe for any blood in the syringe. If blood is observed, remove the syringe immediately, and discard it. Draw up new medication with a new needle and syringe, and repeat the foregoing steps, as needed.

    Ensures that needle is not within a blood vessel.

11. If no blood appears in the syringe, slowly inject the medication.

12. Withdraw the syringe and needle

Table 12.16. *(cont.)*

NURSING ACTIONS	RATIONALE
quickly, at the same angle at which it was inserted.	
13. Apply slight pressure to the site, with a sterile 2 × 2 gauze pad; gently massage the muscle, if indicated.	Prevents medication from leaking at the site; increases circulation and enhances absorption.
14. Apply Band-Aid™.	Keeps the site clean and dry.
15. Comfort and praise the child after administration.	Decreases traumatic effects of the procedure.
a. *Infants*—offer a pacifier and hold the infant.	
b. *Toddlers/preschoolers*—hold the child close, while the child cries; optional—give a cartoon Band-Aid™ or sticker after the procedure.	
c. *School-age children*—hold the child, if he or she desires; offer a cartoon Band-Aid™ or sticker as a reward for being cooperative.	
d. *Adolescents*—Encourage verbalization of feelings.	
16. Wash your hands.	
17. Document the medication administered, including the site, the dosage of medication, the time it was administered, how the child tolerated the procedure, and any changes in the child's condition following the medication administration.	Communicates the nursing interventions and observations to health-care professionals.

ADMINISTRATION OF INTRAVENOUS MEDICATIONS

Indications Medications are administered by the IV route when gastrointestinal accessibility is limited, absorption is impaired, or high levels of the medication in the bloodstream must be achieved rapidly.[5] Some medications cause pain or damage when given by the IM or subcutaneous routes.[9] IV administration (a) provides rapid onset and immediate action, (b) allows continuous administration at an uninterrupted rate,[9] and (c) allows for immediate termination of the medication if a complication arises.[9]

Contraindications An IV site that is questionably patent; medications that are not made for IV use or for which the child has a known sensitivity.

Complications Extravasation of medication into tissue; adverse reaction to medication; vascular irritation;[9] speed shock.[9]

Equipment

Medication (for IV administration only)
Infusate and buretrol™
Alcohol wipes
Povidone–iodine wipes (for immunosuppressed child)
Flush syringe of NSS
1-cc heparin flush syringe (10 units of heparin/cc)
Syringe and needle or commercially available needleless port system

Psychosocial Considerations   After the child has an IV line in place, he or she may become frightened at the sight of another needle. Explain to the child that the needle goes into the IV tubing and not into her or him.

Nursing responsibilities are described in Tables 12.17, 12.18, and 12.19.

Table 12.17. Nursing Responsibilities

NURSING ACTIONS	RATIONALE
1. Check the medication order for the dosage, amount, time, and route. Check the child's ED identification band; assess for any medication allergies.	Ensures the proper administration of the medication to the correct child.
2. Check medication references for the rate of administration, the compatibility of the medication with the diluent, and the amount of diluent; observe the medication for precipitate.	
3. Wash your hands.	
4. Explain to the child and the family the need for the IV medication.	Enhances their understanding and cooperation.
5. Clean the insertion site with alcohol, and check the patency of the IV by slowly and gently aspirating the syringe, while checking for a blood return. If no blood return is visible, slowly administer NSS, and check for the ease of flow or extravasation into the subcutaneous tissue.	Avoids extravasation of medication into tissues.
6. Administer the medication by IV push or IV drip, as appropriate (see Tables 12.18 and 12.19).	
7. Resume IV fluids, as ordered, or flush with heparin solution if IV is for intermittent use only.	Provides patency of IV site.
8. Praise the child for cooperating; wash your hands.	
9. Document the time, dosage, and amount of medication, and the flush administered, how the child toler-	Communicates the nursing interventions and observations to health-care professionals.

Table 12.17. *(cont.)*

NURSING ACTIONS	RATIONALE
ated the medication administration, as well as any changes in the child's condition.	

Table 12.18. IV Push

NURSING ACTIONS	RATIONALE
1. Clean the insertion site with alcohol; use povidone–iodine followed by alcohol for immunosuppressed children.	Prevents contamination of the IV line.
2. Administer the medication, as directed, over the recommended time, through the closest insertion site to the child.	Allows for rapid absorption of medication.
3. Wipe the hub with alcohol, and slowly flush with $1/2$–1 cc of NSS flush.	Ensures administration of the entire dose of ordered medication.
4. If the IV is for intermittent use, flush it with 1-cc of heparin (10 units of heparin/1-cc).[3]	

Table 12.19. IV Drip

NURSING ACTIONS	RATIONALE
1. Clean the insertion site with alcohol; use povidone–iodine and alcohol for immunosuppressed children.	Prevents contamination of the IV line.
2. Place the medication in a buretrol™ with the minimum amount of recommended diluent. Place the IV tubing on an infusion pump, if indicated.	
3. After the medication is infused, add approximately 10 cc or more of maintenance fluid into the buretrol™ to flush the medication through the IV tubing.	Ensures that all medication has been infused.

MEDICATION ADMINISTRATION VIA CENTRAL VENOUS ACCESS DEVICE

Partially Implanted Venous Access Devices

Indications Partially implanted venous access devices are indicated for children who require prolonged or frequent venous access and when peripheral access is unobtainable in children with chronic illnesses who require frequent medications, parenteral nutrition, blood transfusions, or repeated blood sampling. There are two types of catheters: tunneled and nontunneled. The administration of medications is similar with both types of catheters

In *nontunneled catheters,* the proximal tip of the catheter is threaded internally to a major blood vessel, and the distal end is sutured in place at the exit site on the skin. This type of catheter is usually indicated for short-term use. Examples of these catheters by brand are Arrow, Cook, and Acute Care Groshong®.

Tunneled catheters are usually inserted surgically. The proximal end of the catheter sits in a major blood vessel, with the distal end tunneled from the entrance site in the vessel through the subcutaneous fascia of the chest or abdominal wall (see Figure 12.5). It is brought up through the exit site on the chest or abdomen. This type of catheter has a Dacron® polyester fiber cuff(s) approximately 2 cm from the exit site on the trunk. The cuff(s) are in the subcutaneous fascia, which promotes fibrin growth around the cuff, to help anchor the catheter in place. The cuff(s) can also prevent bacteria from migrating up the catheter.[6] Examples of these catheters by trade name are Broviac®, Hickman®, Raff®, Corcath®, Groshong®, Quinton®.[10]

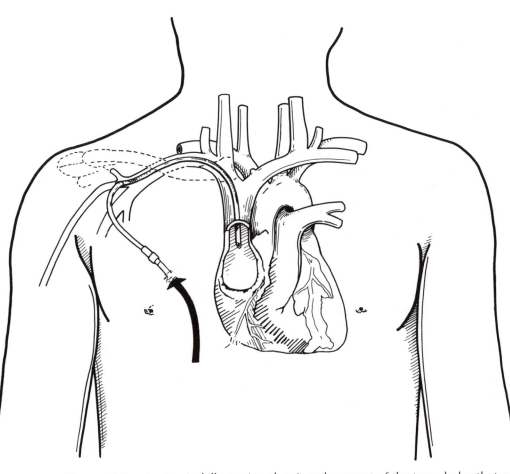

Figure 12.5.   Anatomical illustration showing placement of the tunneled catheter.

Contraindications Open wounds at the insertion site. Edema, redness, or skin irritation at the tunnel tract and/or skin site.

Complications Air emboli; sepsis/infection; dislodgement of catheter, causing extravasation into tissue; perforation of vessel; occlusion from clot formation; cardiac perforation; pneumothorax.[10]

Equipment

> Medication
> Sterile gloves
> 2-cc sterile NSS flush syringe[11]
> 1-cc sterile heparinized flush syringe (100 units heparin/1 cc)[11]
> Nonserrated hemostats or catheter clamp
> Two 3-cc syringes
> Alcohol wipes
> Povidone–iodine wipes
> Rubber-hubbed cap or commercially available needleless port system

Psychosocial Considerations Encouragement and reassurance should be given throughout the procedure. Parents may have concerns about the nurse's ability to access these devices, as they may be used to the techniques of acute care or home care nurses. In particular, the parents may fear infection or readmission for placement of another device. The emergency nurse should reassure the parent that the proper aseptic technique will be used. If the emergency nurse has difficulty or is unfamiliar with accessing the device, assistance from the parent or another nurse proficient in the technique should be sought.

Nursing responsibilities are described in Table 12.20.

Table 12.20. Nursing Responsibilities

NURSING ACTIONS	RATIONALE
1. Check the medication order for the dosage, amount, time, and route. Check the child's ED identification band; assess for any medication allergies.	Ensures proper administration of medication to the correct child.
2. Explain to the child and the family the need for the medication.	Enhances their understanding and cooperation.
3. Wash your hands; don sterile gloves.	
4. For tunneled catheters, palpate the catheter through its tunnel, and feel for the cuff.	Ensures proper catheter placement.
5. Aseptically prepare the medication, NSS flush syringe, and heparinized syringe.	Assists in prevention of line infection.
6. Clamp the catheter with nonserrated hemostats or the appropriate catheter clamp.	Serrated edges may cut or crack the line tubing.
7. Clean the connection between the catheter and the cap twice with povidone–iodine. Let dry.[10]	Decreases risk of infection.

Table 12.20.   (cont.)

NURSING ACTIONS	RATIONALE
8. Disconnect the cap, and attach the NSS syringe; unclamp the catheter.	
9. For nontunneled catheters, gently aspirate for a blood return. For tunneled catheters, do not aspirate.	Checks placement of the nontunneled catheter. Tunneled catheters are very pliable and collapse when aspirated; no blood return is expected.
10. Slowly administer the 2-cc NSS flush or the amount recommended by your institution.	Checks patency of the catheter.
11. Clamp the catheter.	
12. Disconnect the NSS flush syringe, and attach the medication to be administered. Unclamp the catheter, and administer the medication as ordered.	
13. Clamp the catheter, and attach the recommended amount of NSS flush solution, as per institutional policy.	
14. Unclamp the catheter, and administer the NSS flush solution.	Clears the line of any medication.
15. Clamp the catheter. Either attach the IV solution, or attach the heparinized flush syringe if the catheter is for intermittent use.	
16. Unclamp the catheter, and continue the IV administration, as indicated, for intermittent use, clamp the catheter and attach the heparin flush syringe. Unclamp the catheter and flush with the heparin solution. Clamp the catheter, remove the syringe and attach the flushed rubber-hubbed cap. Unclamp the catheter. Be careful not to insert air bubbles while flushing the catheter.	Diminishes the insertion of air bubbles in the line. The heparin flush solution keeps the catheter patent in between uses.
17. Document the medication administered, and its dosage, the amount of flush solution administered, and the amount of heparin administered. Document the appearance and intactness of the catheter and site and the child's response to the medication.	Communicates the nursing interventions and observations to health-care professionals.

TOTALLY IMPLANTED VENOUS ACCESS DEVICES

Indications   The totally implanted venous access device is indicated for long-term use. This catheter is surgically placed into a vessel, body cavity, or organ and then attached to a reservoir. The reservoir is placed under the skin in the subcutaneous tissue. A rubber septum covers the reservoir of the port, so that medications or fluid can be administered. The port is completely covered by the skin; all that is seen is a slight bulge. Children tend to favor this type of catheter because there are slight changes (bulge) in body appearance, dressing changes are not required, and the catheter cannot be pulled out.[6] This type of device has a reduced risk of infection, and when not in use, it only requires a monthly heparin flush.[6] Examples of such catheters by trade name are Mediport, Infusaport®, Porta-cath®, Hickman®, Davol®[10] (see Figure 12.6).

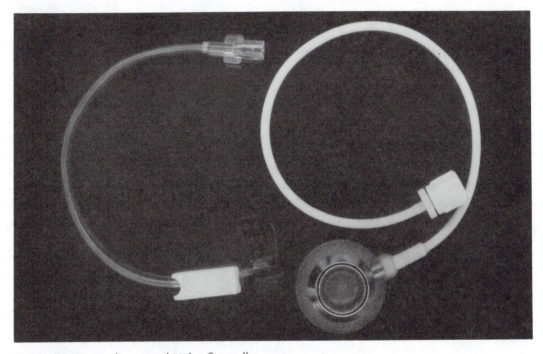

Figure 12.6.   Mediport and Huber® needle.

Contraindications   Open wounds near the reservoir. Edema or redness near the port; known sensitivity to the medication.

Complications   Infection, occlusion, accidental removal or displacement; cardiac tamponade; air embolism; extravasation into the tissue if the needle is not in the correct position.

Equipment

> Correct needle size and type
> Noncoring Huber® point needles (see Figure 12.6)
> A ³/₄" 22-gauge 90-degree bent-angle needle is most often used
> A ¹/₂" needle may be used on very thin children
> A 1" needle may be used on children with a very thick layer of tissue over the
>   port.

A straight-angle needle is used for parallel ports
Medication, as ordered
Sterile gloves
2.5–3-cc sterile heparin flush syringe (100 units/cc)[3]
1–5-cc NSS flush
2–10-cc NSS flush syringe
Sterile towel or drape
3-Povidone–iodine wipes
Povidone–iodine ointment
Band-Aid™
Two 3-cc and one 20-cc syringes
For infusion, add:
   Transparent dressing
   Two 2 × 2 gauze pads
   Tape or Steri-strips®
   Rubber-hubbed cap or needleless port system

Psychosocial Considerations   After multiple insertions, the site becomes cal-
loused, and less discomfort is experienced. Encouragement and reassurance
should be given throughout the procedure. The parents may have concerns
about the emergency nurse's ability to access these devices, as they are familiar
with the techniques of acute care or home care nurses. The parents may fear
infection or readmission for placement of another device. The emergency
nurse should reassure the parent that the proper aseptic technique will be
used. If the emergency nurse has difficulty or is unfamiliar with accessing the
device, assistance from the parent or another nurse proficient in the technique should be sought.
   Nursing responsibilities are described in Table 12.21.

Table 12.21. Nursing Responsibilities

NURSING ACTIONS	RATIONALE
1. Explain to the child and the family the need for the medication.	Enhances their understanding and cooperation.
2. Identify the septum by palpating the outer perimeters of the port.	Confirms insertion location.
3. Wash your hands; observe for any swelling or redness at the site.	
4. Aseptically assemble and prime the IV tubing and/or medication sy- ringe, the NSS flushes, and the hep- arin flush. Place these supplies on a sterile towel.	Decreases the risk of infection; al- lows sterile field for supplies.
5. Don gloves, and maintain strict aseptic technique.	Reduces the risk of infection.
6. Prime the needle and the tubing connector with NSS. Keep the sy- ringe attached, and clamp the tub- ing. If blood is to be drawn, do not prime needle and tubing; attach a dry syringe.	Checks the patency of the needle and flushes air from the tubing.

Table 12.21.   (*cont.*)

NURSING ACTIONS	RATIONALE
7. Instruct the child to lie in a supine position; another person may be necessary to assist in positioning the child.	Assists in proper access to the port.
8. Cleanse the skin with povidone–iodine and allow to dry.	Disinfects the skin.
9. Place a sterile drape around the insertion site.	Reduces the risk of contamination.
10. Locate the area on the skin where the port diaphragm is located; position the port between two fingers.	Keeps the port in position.
11. At a 90-degree angle, firmly push the noncoring needle into the port, just until you feel the needle tip touch the hard back of the port[10] (see Figure 12.7).	Ensures proper needle insertion.

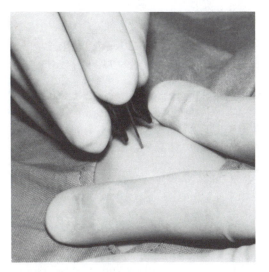

Figure 12.7.   Insertion of Huber needle into Mediport.

12. Aspirate slightly checking for a blood return. Slowly inject 2–3 cc of NSS,[11] or slowly aspirate the amount of blood needed for testing. For administering bolus medication, or continuous infusion, see Steps 13 and 14. For discontinuing the medication or infusion, see step 15.	Validates catheter placement in the vessel.
13. *For bolus/intermittent medication administration:*	
a. Clamp the tubing attached to the	

Table 12.21.   (*cont.*)

NURSING ACTIONS	RATIONALE
Huber® needle and attach the NSS flush syringe.	
b. Unclamp the tubing and slowly inject 10 cc of the NSS flush. (Amount may vary with child's size and fluid status.)[3] Observe for redness or edema near the insertion site.	Ensures that the needle is in the port and not the tissue.
c. Clamp the tubing attach the medication syringe.	
d. Unclamp the tubing and administer the medication, as ordered.	
14. *For continuous infusion:*	
a. Apply a small amount of povidone ointment to the insertion site, and stabilize the needle in place with Steri-strip®s or tape and support with 2 × 2 gauze pads (see Figure 12.8a).	Helps prevent needle from slipping out of port during infusion.
b. Apply a transparent dressing without applying tension on the tubing (see Figure 12.8b).	Decreases the tension on the line and keeps the insertion site clean.
c. Clamp the tubing and attach the primed IV tubing. Unclamp, and begin the infusion as ordered.	Decreases risk of infection to the catheter.
15. *Discontinuing the medication or infusion:*	
a. Clamp the tubing and attach an NSS syringe. Unclamp the tubing, then flush the port with 10 cc NSS flush.	Clears the line of any medications.
b. Clamp the tubing and attach the heparin syringe. Unclamp the tubing and flush with the heparin flush solution as you withdraw the needle.[3]	This flush fills the dead space with heparin and creates a positive pressure in the line, thereby maintaining catheter potency.
c. Hold light pressure on the insertion site with sterile gauze for a few seconds. Apply a small amount of povidone–iodine ointment and a Band-Aid™.	The needle may cause a puncture opening in the skin; covering it may decrease risk of infection.
d. Document the accessing procedure and the medications administered. Include the intactness of the needle, and the amount of flush solution instilled, as well as the child's tolerance of the procedure.	Communicates the nursing interventions and observations to health-care professionals.

Table 12.21.   *(cont.)*

NURSING ACTIONS	RATIONALE

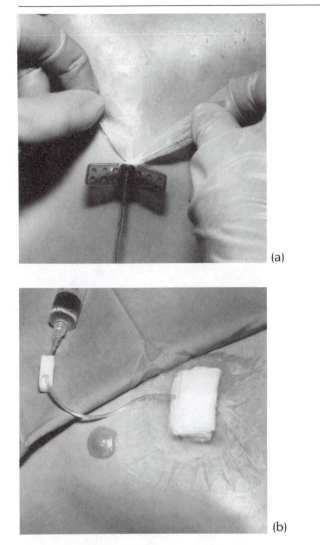

(a)

(b)

Figure 12.8. Securing the Huber® needle during infusion: **(a)** stabilizing the needle, and **(b)** supporting it with gauze pads.

REFERENCES

1. Kelley S. Ed. Pediatric emergency nursing. Norwalk, CT: Appleton & Lange, 1988;138, 225, 362.
2. Whaley L & Wong D. Clinical manual of pediatric nursing. 3rd ed. St. Louis: CV Mosby Co., 1990;555, 565.
3. Skale N. Manual of pediatric nursing procedures. Philadelphia: JB Lippincott Co., 1992;123, 126–127, 342, 816, 817.
4. Howry L. Pediatric medications. Philadelphia: JB Lippincott Co., 1981;53, 55.

5. Whaley L., Wong L. Nursing care of infants and children. 4th ed. St. Louis: Mosby-Yearbook Co., 1991;1229–1232, 1235–1236.
6. Whaley L., Wong D. Essentials of nursing care. 2nd ed. St. Louis: CV Mosby Co., 1985;566–567, 559.
7. Servonsky J., Opas SR. Nursing management of children. Boston: Jones & Bartlett, 1987;813.
8. Hughes W., Bueschler E. Pediatric procedures. 2nd ed. Philadelphia: WB Saunders Co., 1980;154–155, 263–264.
9. Plumer AL. Principles and practice of intravenous therapy. 4th ed. Boston: Little, Brown & Co., 1987;371–372.
10. Blumer J. A practical guide to pediatric intensive care. 3rd ed. St. Louis: Mosby-Yearbook, 1990;870–875.
11. Hazinski MF. Ed. Nursing care of the critically ill child. 2nd ed. St. Louis: Mosby-Yearbook, 1992;1076–1077.

13

Procedures for the Collection of Evidence in Physical and Sexual Abuse of Children

Bonnie Clemence and Marianne Bove

OVERVIEW OF CHILD ABUSE

The incidence of child abuse has reached staggering proportions. For this reason, it is imperative that the emergency nurse be able to recognize the factors that heighten concern about suspected child abuse and neglect. The law requires that any suspicion of child abuse or neglect must be reported to the appropriate agency; the law also grants immunity from liability to individuals who report their concerns in good faith. Specifications for reporting and documenting abuse vary from state to state; consult your local child protective agency to learn about the proper procedure for reporting abuse.

Abuse can be categorized as physical abuse or neglect, emotional abuse and neglect, or sexual abuse. Tables 13.1 through 13.4 illustrate how to recognize the "red flags" of abuse in children and families.

Table 13.1. Parent and Child Risk Factors for Abuse[1]

PARENT RISK FACTORS	CHILD RISK FACTORS
Isolated, poorly socialized—often overwhelmed and/or depressed.	Infants separated from mother at birth because of illness or prematurity.
Parents were abused themselves as children.	Children with impulse disorders or behavioral problems.
Single parents.	Foster children.
Poor ability of the parents to deal with anger, stress, frustration. Recent severe family stress or loss.	Child who is perceived by the parents as difficult or bad.

Table 13.1.   *(cont.)*

Psychotic, alcoholic, or addicted parents.
Unrealistic expectations of child and/or perceived inability of the child to meet parental expectations.

Table 13.2.   Characteristics of Child Abuse from the History[2]

History given by parent is inconsistent with existing injury.
Absence of any history of or explanation for injury.
Parent reluctant to give information.
Child is developmentally incapable of the specific self-injury.
Delay in seeking medical care.
Inconsistencies or changes in the history.
History of repeated injuries or hospitalizations.
Inappropriate response to the severity of the injury.

Reprinted by permission from SJ Kelley, *Pediatric Emergency Nursing.* East Norwalk, CT: Appleton & Lange, p. 5.

Table 13.3.   Characteristics of Physical Abuse on Examination

Integumentary
   Bruises found in unusual locations,[1] such as back, upper arms, buttocks, thighs, face, hands, ears, or feet.
   Multiple bruises in different stages of healing
   Skin injuries in a configuration that suggests use of a weapon (e.g., looped cord)
   Immersion burns
   Cigarette burns—8–10 mm in diameter and indurated at the margin[2]
   Contact burns in the pattern of a hot object (iron, electric stove burner)
   Human bites—when the diameter is measured and is comparable to an adult mouth
   Traction alopecia
Musculoskeletal
   Multiple fractures at various stages of healing
   Metaphyseal fractures
   Long-bone fractures or rib fractures
Central Nervous System
   Skull fracture without adequate explanation
   Shake injuries: cervical subluxation; retinal hemorrhages; subdural hemorrhage; brain contusion
Gastrointestinal System
   Ruptured spleen
   Lacerated liver
   Duodenal hematoma
   Intestinal and mesenteric tears
   Abdominal pain, distention, tenderness, and vomiting

Table 13.3.   (*cont.*)

Cardiopulmonary
   Pulmonary or cardiac contusion
   Hemothorax
   Pneumothorax

Table 13.4.   Psychosocial Indicators of Abuse

PHYSICAL ABUSE	NEGLECT	EMOTIONAL ABUSE
Extreme withdrawal[2]	Developmental delay[2]	Excessively passive or aggressive[2]
Indiscriminate friendliness or inappropriate display of affection[2]	Malnutrition[2]	Obsessive–compulsive disorders[2]
	Lethargy	
	Excessively passive[2]	Substance abuse[2]
Appearance of being frightened of parents and of going home[2]	Failure to thrive[2]	Runaway behavior[2]
	Frequent truancy	
Inappropriate reactions following painful procedures[2]		
Apprehensiveness when other children are crying[2]		

Table 13.5.   Nursing Responsibilities in Suspected Child Physical Abuse

NURSING ACTIONS	RATIONALE
1. Obtain a history from the parents and the child, whenever possible. Include past medical history and psychosocial history. Maintain a nonjudgmental attitude and offer open-ended questions.	Promotes an objective assessment of the situation.
2. Obtain medical records.	May indicate a prior history of abuse or may verify the history obtained.
3. Perform a head-to-toe physical assessment. *Note:* When the child presents with a life-threatening condition or significant trauma, stabilization of airway, breathing, and circulation take immediate priority.	Initial goal is to stabilize the child.
4. Obtain laboratory and radiographic studies, as indicated by the situation and the physician's orders.	Assists in differential diagnosis.
5. Collaborate with other health-care professionals (e.g., ED physician, nurse, social worker).	Facilitates optimal management of the family in crisis.

Table 13.5. *(cont.)*

NURSING ACTIONS	RATIONALE
6. Report suspected abuse to child protection agency, social services, or local police, for either further investigation or placement of the child who is at immediate risk.	Fosters the well-being of the child and family.
7. Notify parents of your report of suspicions. Offer empathy and emotional support in your explanations. Emphasis should be placed on concern for the child's safety and how the family may be best helped.	Promotes understanding of why this situation is being reported.
8. Document your findings.	Provides medical and legal records.
a. Complete appropriate forms, as required by individual state laws. Some states may require sketches or drawings of injuries on a body chart.	
b. Describe in detail each bruise, lesion, or burn, according to size, location, color, and shape.[2]	
c. All significant statements by both parent(s) and child should be carefully recorded, using as many direct quotes as possible.[2]	
d. Include a description of the behaviors of both parent and child.[2]	
e. Obtain color Polaroid photographs of the injuries. Parental consent for photographing may be required in some states.[2]	
9. Arrange for follow-up intervention with a child protective agency, social services, or family-in-crisis services.	Provides support to the child and family.

COLLECTION OF EVIDENCE FOR SEXUAL ABUSE

Indications   An assessment, including collection of evidence, should be initiated whenever sexual abuse is suspected.

Contraindications   None.

Complications   Inadmissible evidence if the specimens are incorrectly obtained and processed.

Equipment

>   Sex crime kit
>   Labels for specimens
>   Brown paper bag
>   Phlebotomy equipment

Psychosocial Considerations   Assisting with the collection of evidence for suspected sexual abuse is emotionally wrenching for all involved parties—the child, the family, and the nurses and physicians. While a brief overview of psychosocial considerations is presented here, further information can be obtained from the cited references regarding child physical and sexual abuse.

Infants and young toddlers are unable to verbalize the abusive incidents, but they may exhibit behavioral and physical changes consistent with sexual abuse. Older toddlers and preschoolers may be either afraid or unable to verbalize what has happened to them. Giving them either crayons and paper or dolls may allow them to express themselves more readily. Children in this age group are often preoccupied with their private parts and may feel worried about what happened to them. They may have been threatened by the perpetrator and may be afraid to tell about the perpetrator's actions.

School-age children may also be reluctant to tell about what has happened to them for fear of retribution or embarrassment. Adolescents may be afraid—especially in cases of rape (including date rape) or incest—or have low self-esteem (if the abuse has occurred over a period of time). Adolescents occasionally present with a suicide attempt, and the sexual abuse may be discovered at that time.

Some general considerations in approaching children with suspected sexual abuse are as follows:[1]

> Provide a calm, relaxed, and nonjudgmental atmosphere; continue to offer reassurance and empathy throughout the process.
>
> Avoid asking leading questions; write down the child's direct quotes.
>
> If the parents are supportive and calm, it can be helpful to have them present during the interview and examination. If the parents are not calm or supportive, or if the child seems reticent in their presence, a nurse, social worker, or other appropriately designated person should provide support for the child; interviews of the parent and child should be conducted separately. An adolescent should be permitted to choose whomever he or she wishes to be present for the exam, such as a friend or parent.
>
> If the child is unwilling to talk, defer the interview for a return visit or for a play session with an experienced health-care professional.

To help the child discuss the incident, the nurse should:

1. Establish rapport and gain the child's trust by discussing nonthreatening topics, such as school friends, interests, hobbies.
2. Address the subject at hand, by saying, "Sometimes, children we see who have (chief complaint) are worried because someone is making them do scary or upsetting things or is touching them in places that they shouldn't, or even is doing things that hurt them. People who do these things have a problem and need help, but the only way for them to get help is if children tell someone else. Could this be happening to you?"[1]
3. Establish a common vocabulary with younger children, who may not understand the words "penis" and "vagina."[3]
4. Praise the child for sharing information with you and for cooperating with the examination.

Nursing responsibilities are described in Table 13.6.

Table 13.6. Nursing Responsibilities

NURSING ACTIONS	RATIONALE
1. Explain to the child and the family the need for the procedure. Explain each step as it happens.	Enhances their understanding and cooperation.
2. Assess the child's emotional status. If the child is uncooperative or distressed, either defer the examination or complete the exam under general anesthesia. Do *not* restrain the child.[4]	Prevents further emotional trauma.[4]
3. Assess the need for additional emotional support (pastoral care, social worker, sexual assault advocate, or additional nurse). One nurse should follow through with the ED visit from beginning to end. The physician and nurse should examine the child together.	Having one nurse protects the chain of evidence, prevents the child from being examined more than once, allows for a witness to be present, and provides consistent emotional support.
4. Gather a history of the event, preferably in the child's own words. Document the child's words in quotations.	Physical findings substantiate the child's allegations.
5. Allow the child to draw on paper the history of events or use anatomically correct dolls to demonstrate what has occurred.	Illustrating the event may be less traumatic than verbalizing the event for some children.
6. The history should include the following: a. Who: alleged perpetrator(s) b. When: time(s) and date(s) of event(s) c. Where: location of event(s) d. What happened (see Item 5) e. Activities since the event (bathing, douching, urination, defecation, and change of clothing)	Physical findings substantiate the child's allegations.
7. If the child presents to the ED wearing clothing that was worn during the assault, place the clothing in a brown paper bag.[4] Label each item, and seal the bag.	Plastic bags can cause chemical changes.[4] Labeling ensures proper identification.
8. If the assault is recent and the child describes a struggle that ensued, obtain nail clippings and scrapings from under the child's fingernails. Place these in an envelope, and label them.[4]	Serves as a source of identification.

Table 13.6.   (*cont.*)

NURSING ACTIONS	RATIONALE
9. If the assault was recent and if appropriate, comb the child's pubic hair for the assailant's hair; place them in an envelope, and label it "pubic hair combing." Use tweezers to pluck pubic hairs from the child (if applicable); place them in a separate envelope, and label it "pubic hair pluckings."[4]	Serves as a control for identification.
10. If the sexual abuse was recent, use a Wood's lamp to examine the child's perineum, perianal region, abdomen, and thighs;[2] consider doing a head-to-toe exam with the Wood's lamp. Follow Step 11 for a female or 12 for a male, then proceed to Step 13.	Detects the presence of dried semen.
11. *Examination of a female*	
a. Position the child:	
(1) *Prepubertal*—Place the child on the parent's lap in a frogleg position (see Figure 13.1). If the child is able, ask her to hold her labia majora apart.[4]	Allows child some control over procedure.
(2) *Prepubescent*—The child can be placed on a table in the knee–chest position.[4]	Allows for visualization of the perineum.
b. If an internal examination is needed, a pediatric speculum, nasal speculum, or pediatric laryngoscope should be used.[4]	
c. Observe for the condition of the hymenal ring, bruising, bleeding, and lacerations, to the genitalia and rectum.[4]	
12. *Examination of a male*	
a. Place the child in a lateral decubitus position.	
b. Observe for bleeding, bruising, and lacerations to the genitalia and anus.[4]	
13. If the assault is recent (within 72 hours), secretions from the vagina and rectum should be examined for the presence of sperm or semen.	Identifies recent assault. Motile and non-motile sperm are identified using a "wet preparation" in which the secretions are mixed with saline on a slide and examined under a microscope. Semen are detected by allow-

Table 13.6. *(cont.)*

NURSING ACTIONS	RATIONALE

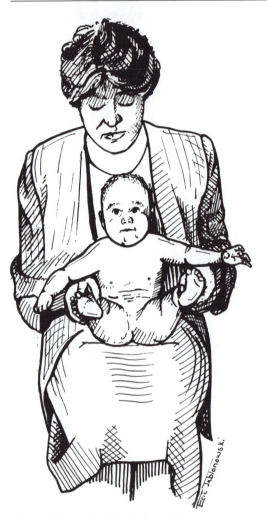

Figure 13.1. Method of positioning a young child for a genital examination when sexual abuse is suspected. The examination may be less traumatic if completed with the child sitting on the mother's lap. The mother can hold the child in a frogleg position to facilitate the exam.

14. Obtain cultures (gonococcal, chlamydial) from the throat, rectum, vagina, and male urethra; repeat this procedure in 7 days.

15. Perform a human chorionic gonadotropin (HCG) serum pregnancy test

ing secretions to air dry on a slide and testing with acid phosphatase.

All areas are cultured because the child may minimize types of sexual activity due to fear or embarrassment.[4]

Serves as baseline data.

Table 13.6. (*cont.*)

NURSING ACTIONS	RATIONALE
in females who are postmenarchal. Repeat the test in 6 weeks if negative.[4]	
16. Obtain Venereal Disease Research Laboratories (VDRL) specimen; repeat in 6–8 weeks.[4] Consider obtaining a blood sample for HIV testing.	Serves as baseline data. Follow up should include HIV testing in 6 months.
17. Administer antibiotics if ordered by the physician.	Initiates therapy in the event of sexually transmitted disease (STD).
18. Administer a postcoital oral contraceptive to a female at risk for pregnancy, if ordered by the physician.	Prevents pregnancy.
19. Report sexual abuse to the appropriate agency.	Nurses, like all health-care professionals, are mandated by law to report sexual abuse.
20. Keep specimens in the possession of appropriate health-care professionals until the legal authorities arrive.	Prevents tampering with the evidence obtained.
21. If the child's clothing is kept for evidence, obtain clothing for the child to wear home.	
22. Document the time of specimen collection, how the child tolerated the procedure, who obtained the evidence, and when it was given to the police, as well as follow-up services for the family.	Ensures movement from health-care professionals to the police, to preserve the chain of evidence that will allow verification of materials in court.[3]
23. Refer the child and family for counseling.	Provides continuity and provides the child and family with opportunities to discuss their fears and concerns.

REFERENCES

1. Davis HW, Hughes SE. Suspected child abuse and neglect. 5th ed. The Children's Hospital of Pittsburgh SCAN Program. Pittsburgh: Department of Pediatrics, University of Pittsburgh; Department of Clinical Social Work, Children's Hospital of Pittsburgh, 1985;7–10.
2. Kelley SJ. Child abuse and neglect. In: Kelley SJ, ed. Pediatric emergency nursing. E. Norwalk, CT: Appleton & Lange, 1988;8,14–15, 18–19.
3. Ludwig S. Child abuse. In: Fleisher GR, Ludwig S, eds. Textbook of pediatric emergency medicine. 2nd ed. Baltimore: Williams & Wilkins, 1988;1147,1157.
4. Kelley SJ. Sexual abuse of children. In: Kelley SJ, ed. Pediatric emergency nursing. E. Norwalk, CT: Appleton & Lange, 1988;41–43,47–48.

Index

NOTE: Page numbers in parentheses indicate illustrations.